What people are s [barcode: C000027434]

This One is Special

A powerful and very personal story of courage and kindness, lived every day. I admire this family so much.
Bear Grylls, adventurer, global TV personality, best-selling author and World Scout Chief Ambassador

Wow, I was so moved by this story.
Anita Moorjani, international speaker and the author of *New York Times* best-seller *Dying To Be Me*

I stayed up far too long last night reading *This One is Special* from start to finish. I love it. It is like a cool, clear, endless glass of water on a warm summer's day – it has such clarity and depth.
Gillian Clark, Chair of The Healing Trust

A radiant and inspiring story of how to make happiness out of adversity – by having faith in goodness, learning from dreams, and trusting in intuition.
Adrian Poole, Fellow in English, Trinity College, Cambridge

This book perfectly captures the conflict between one's own positive views of one's disabled child and the defeatist attitude of professionals. It's life affirming to see how Tim progresses as Suzanne begins to trust her instincts, her dreams and, most of all, her son.
James Melville-Ross, author of *Two for Joy* and *ambassador for Scope*

This One is Special

When your child has a condition that can't be cured, where do you look for answers?

This One
is Special

When your child has a condition that
can't be cured, where do you look for
answers?

Suzanne Askham

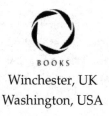

BOOKS
Winchester, UK
Washington, USA

JOHN HUNT PUBLISHING

First published by O-Books, 2020
O-Books is an imprint of John Hunt Publishing Ltd., 3 East St., Alresford,
Hampshire SO24 9EE, UK
office@jhpbooks.com
www.johnhuntpublishing.com
www.o-books.com

For distributor details and how to order please visit the 'Ordering' section on our website.

ISBN: 978 1 78904 317 4
978 1 78904 318 1 (ebook)
Library of Congress Control Number: 2019931139

A CIP catalogue record for this book is available from the British Library.

Design: Stuart Davies

UK: Printed and bound by CPI Group (UK) Ltd, Croydon, CR0 4YY
US: Printed and bound by Thomson-Shore, 7300 West Joy Road, Dexter, MI 48130

We operate a distinctive and ethical publishing philosophy in
all areas of our business, from our global network of authors to
production and worldwide distribution.

Contents

For Tim and Grace, with love

Previous books by the author

Coping when Your Child has Special Needs, ISBN 0-85969-825-4, Sheldon Press, 2000

Adventure Unlimited: Living and Working Abroad, ISBN 1-85340-270-2, Piccadilly Press, 1993

Acknowledgements

They say it takes a village to raise a child. In our case, it took an extended community spread across several countries and two continents to raise our son Tim. His complex learning and physical disabilities have resulted in countless people helping him, and us. From friends, family and neighbours to teachers and medical staff, we are grateful to every single one of them. Many of these individuals are acknowledged within the book. There are many others who have helped us since, some of whom are included here.

Warm appreciation is due to all the staff of National Star College, near Cheltenham, including Adam Jones and Hayley Phelps; the incomparable Di Knight (thank you for all the amazing adventures), kindly Bonni Hopkins and the many other highly enabling carers; tutors including Jill Willingham, and learning mentors including Dave Hansell; Katherine Rowland and the nursing team, as well as many empowering therapists including Heather Cater and Dan Freeth; not to mention the students who help to give the college such a buzz and make it an outstanding place for all like Tim to live and study.

Respect and gratitude are due to the many health professionals who between them have saved Tim's life and enabled him to thrive. Thank you, Dr Mark Juniper, for not giving up on our son and open-mindedly looking beyond diagnoses to encourage Tim's individual potential. Thanks also to your colleagues and all the incredible staff at ICU, Great Western Hospital, Swindon, as well as respiratory specialist Sam Backway and her colleagues in the sleep unit. Much appreciation is due to community nurses Penny Keepence and Richard James, and physio Kim Dempsey – Tim's amazing cycling records on his gym bike would not have happened without you! Peter Cockhill of Stillpoint in Bath, I am so grateful to you, for helping both Tim and myself over many years.

Thank you to Tim's entire care team – from Alexandros Chantzopoulos, Gabriel Bratescu, Esther Boyer and colleagues, to the indefatigable office staff including Celia Rodrigues, you are much appreciated. Suzie Gardner, Julie Welsh and Charlotte Drinkwater, you are the dream team. I hope you know how much Tim loves all the adventures you take him on, and how much he thrives as a result of them. Andrea Mellors, for all your ongoing support, and rock-steady help in times of crisis, heartfelt thanks. Geraldine Francis and Sue Whelan of Fired Thoughts Arts Studio, the way you have helped Tim to develop personalised ceramic techniques has been much appreciated.

Thank you to those gentle souls who meditate with me, including Sue Cann, Jill Dunnley, Caroline Keevil, Katharina Kronig, Jennie Meek, Diane Ramsay-Arthur, Kerstie Walthall and Jayne White, and all who have come along over the past nine years. I have always appreciated the companionable silence, the authentic conversations, and the insights.

Moving on to the actual writing of *This One is Special*, I'm especially grateful to editor Jennifer Day for sensitive editing and thoughtful validation at a time when I needed it. Thanks are also due to all at John Hunt Publishing. I'm grateful that *This One is Special* has found such a suitable home. Your publishing process is a joy.

Finally, I'd like to thank my much-loved family: our supportive parents; our children, Tim and Grace – you are each a dearly loved hero in your own right; and my cherished partner, Steven, for all the love, adventures and support. As you once unforgettably said to me, *"Dum vivimus vivamus"* – While we live, let us live.

Prologue

I hope you will go out and let stories happen to you, and that you will work them, water them with your blood and tears and your laughter until they bloom, till you yourself burst into bloom. Then you will see what medicines they make, and where and when to apply them. That is the work. The only work.

Clarissa Pinkola Estés, from *Women Who Run With the Wolves*

It's 10pm on a late summer's evening in 2013. I am in our old stone house, in Wiltshire. The children are asleep upstairs, Steven is out at a dinner in London. And I am about to open a time capsule.

I'm nervous. I decide to put off the moment by walking to the fridge and getting out a beer. I open the bottle; toss the metal cap in the recycling caddy. I pour the beer. Without even taking a sip, I put the glass of beer down where I promptly forget about it. I rinse the bottle out, and place that too in the recycling caddy.

My mind is turbulent. I haven't looked at the manuscript of *The Miracle Child* in 15 years. It belongs to a different era. Why mess with it now?

The reason isn't hard to find. Recently I broke a long silence. I wrote a blog post about our 17-year-old disabled son, Tim. I called it, "What I wish I'd told Anita Moorjani", and I posted it on Anita Moorjani's Facebook page. The author of *Dying To Be Me* has a beautiful community there, where people bare their souls. It felt good to do it. I also posted a picture of Tim with his dad, Steven. Choosing that photo made me cry. I knew a door that had been closed for quite some time was being allowed to open. I was allowing it to open.

It's true, I have talked about Tim quite a bit with the wonderful souls who come to my Studio and meditate with me there. I consider myself to be open on the subject. But I have kept the conversations small and private.

When Tim was little, when we were still living in Richmond, I wrote a book called *Coping when Your Child has Special Needs* for Sheldon Press. And at the time of publication there were articles and photos of Tim in one national paper, and a handful of magazines. But I left all that behind when we moved to Wiltshire. Without realising, I became quiet on the subject of our beautiful, mysterious, disabled boy.

So why break the silence now?

"Wow, I was so moved by this blog post!!" wrote Anita Moorjani. "Thank you, Suzanne Askham. Next time, Suzanne, we'll definitely talk more! Sending love and hugs to you and your beautiful son."

After Anita wrote that, my blog was suddenly flooded with visitors. Their comments, shared stories and support were extremely moving to me. And I realised that it might be a good thing to be more open. It might be good for Tim. It might be good for other children and young adults like him. It might help other parents, including us.

But more than that, it might help all who are going through their own particular version of the pain of everyday reality.

Maybe you, reading this, maybe you too have struggled with turbulent events in your own life, or the life of someone you love.

Maybe, just maybe, you have also experienced unexpected moments of bliss.

And maybe you have wondered how to reconcile these two experiences into one life.

That, in a nutshell, is what has happened to me. One morning, out of the blue, I had a mystical experience of unimaginable bliss. I saw the unity of all beings. I *was* the unity of all beings.

A year later, I gave birth to a child with profound health issues. Tim's body and mind were equally affected. There was no obvious diagnosis. Especially in the early years, we met countless doctors. Not one of them could give a good prognosis.

Somehow Tim, his father Steven and I had to live with this reality.

"I don't know how you cope. I couldn't do it." That is possibly the most common reaction we have had from others.

How would *you* answer that?

So that's why in just a few minutes I'm planning to go to the spare bedroom at the far end of the house, lean down into a corner there, by the desk, and pick up a fat package in an old Jiffy bag. It's curious that over all these years, the manuscript has been kept in such an accessible place, yet never looked at.

I wonder what the energy of the package will feel like when I open it. I expect it to be drenched in sadness, and I'm dreading that.

"Why mess with it after all these years?" I think again.

"Why not?" a small inner voice whispers back to me. It feels like the prompting of my soul.

The Miracle Child came about almost by itself. Our good family friend Tessa Phillips, a London-based costume designer, knew a book editor at a big publishing house. She told the book editor about Tim, and the editor asked me to write a book about him. I was even given the title, *The Miracle Child*.

I liked the title. I was worried, though, that Tim and I might not live up to it. He was, after all, profoundly disabled. That wasn't likely to change any time soon, although I secretly hoped. But there was a mysterious potential in his story.

So I wrote the book, and in the process released a lot of anger. There was in me a fierce desire to help our son in whatever ways were possible.

But just as I was finishing an early draft, the book editor left, and the publishing house had no interest in *The Miracle Child*. I think I half-heartedly tried a couple of other publishers, who duly rejected it. Steven and a few friends read the manuscript and made supportive comments. And then, rather embarrassed about the whole thing, I put it to one side.

I figured that the universe had its reasons for arranging that I wrote *The Miracle Child*, and it had its reasons for the book not to be published after all.

Dawning awareness

When I was around nine years old, I remember standing in a long line with my classmates against a wire fence. We were dressed in white Airtex shirts and navy PE skirts. In front of us, our teacher was giving instructions.

The instructions seemed to go on, and on. Just in front of me was a metal post, about shoulder height to me. It was old, and rusting. At the top of the post were two little rusting holes, all cobwebby. The post seemed much more interesting than the teacher's words, so I leaned forward, imperceptibly, to look at it more closely. The pattern of rust was interesting. Maybe there were insects in those holes?

Temporarily forgetting where I was, I stepped forward for a better look. As I was peering into the holes of that post, the teacher suddenly yelled at me:

"Get back in line, Suzanne!"

Blushing red, I stepped hastily back against the wire fencing, and instantly blended with my classmates.

That summarises how I felt for about the first 30 years of my life. Like many children, I had an enquiring mind, and I loved the many insights that came to me. But I was desperate to be part of the crowd, not to stand out in any way at all.

I became very good at telling myself to get back in line.

Having Tim changed that, of course. From the moment we saw his long, thin body and his wise eyes, we could see he was not a conventional baby. And that meant that however hard I tried, I was never going to make it as a conventional mother.

I can't put off this moment any longer. I go up to the spare bedroom, lean down into the corner, pick up the Jiffy bag, and take it back to the living room. I bring the forgotten glass of beer with me. I feel that I'm going to need it.

The house is very quiet. There are no interruptions. There is nothing to stop me facing my past.

I open the envelope. I draw out the manuscript. A floppy disk is in there too. I wonder if I can get it converted into a modern format.

To my surprise, the energy of the manuscript feels quite different to what I expected. The overriding feeling is one of... eagerness. This story is ready to be heard. It's even excited about it. Wahey! It's dancing a jig.

Yes, there is sadness. There were certainly enough tears as I wrote it. But the sheer bouncy energy of my younger self is apparent. There was rocket fuel in my blood at that time.

The Miracle Child reflects a dawning awareness during the first years of Tim's life. There's a lot it misses out. I'm amazed, as I read through the pages, that I don't mention the mystical vision that I experienced in the year before Tim was born. That vision is something I told only a very few people, until I wrote about it for the first time in that recent blog post.

The mystical vision sustained me throughout the hardest times. I am deeply, fundamentally grateful that I experienced it. Despite that, the 35-year-old me believed it was 'woo woo'. It was unthinkable to mention it in print.

The same goes for the healing methods that I was just beginning to explore at that time. When Tim was just a few weeks old, I took him to a healer called Phil Edwardes. I had never had any contact with healing before. Something drew me to it. No doubt I was desperate.

I sat holding Tim in my arms in an upright chair, looking out of a window, overlooking a pond. It was a peaceful scene. Green-topped trees blew gently in the breeze. The ongoing hospital appointments seemed less important in this sanctuary. What came to mind when I thought of them was a sun-baked desert, devoid of life-giving properties. The appointments drained me of my energy. They drained our son of his. This, in comparison, was an oasis. I felt as though I had been parched, and at last could quench my thirst.

Phil Edwardes put his hands on my shoulders, and kept them there. I felt a gentle, unfamiliar warmth along the length of my spine.

I allowed myself to cry.

Correction: I couldn't help but cry.

It seemed to me then that Phil helped Tim. He certainly helped me, as I discovered a few days later.

I was going to weekly post-natal exercise classes at that time. The week before I took Tim to Phil Edwardes, the teacher had come over to me and felt the abdominal muscles, or 'abs', over my post-pregnancy tummy. She told me that they had separated, and it would be quite a while before they joined up in the middle again.

Then I took Tim to Phil, and felt that gentle warmth along my spine.

A few days later, I returned to the post-natal class. The teacher came over and checked my abs again… and again… and again. She was astonished. "I can't understand it," she said. "They've completely healed."

Though I was tempted, I didn't tell her about my visit to the healer. I was used to trying to blend in with the crowd, and I knew healing, like visions, was 'woo woo'.

Today, I would write *The Miracle Child* differently, for sure. But that is not the point. I make a decision. I'm not going to change this manuscript, beyond some polishing, and necessary additions to bring it up to date. I'm just going to publish it, as it is, in its own raw energy.

All I hope is that those who are able to benefit from this book get the opportunity to read it.

Well, that was two weeks ago. A day or two later, I drove into Chippenham, our local town, to post the floppy disc to Martin, a man I'd tracked down who could hopefully retrieve the data on the disc. Martin gave me precise instructions on how to wrap the disc in bubble wrap and then pack it into a box. The gist was that I was to treat it as delicately as an unborn baby.

My nine-year-old daughter, Grace, was sitting in the front beside me, with the box on her lap. "What's in this box, anyway?" she asked.

"Tears," I answered, only half-joking. "It's a box of tears."

For an instant, Grace looked shocked and horrified.

"It's not wet," she protested. "It can't be tears."

And then her cool persona took over. "Get serious, Mummy," she said.

However, I noticed, as we got out of the car, that she was holding the box rather like an unexploded bomb that was about to go off. And when we finally let the box go at the post office, she looked relieved.

I expected the data to be retrieved pretty well straight away. Martin said he'd email it to me. But we talked yesterday on the phone and it turned out that he's been having problems with it. So far he's retrieved... a big, fat, nothing.

The delay has caused me to change my plans. My first plan was to get the text out as an e-book, in a few days flat.

In the enforced delay, I've been remembering things I left out.

At key times, I have seen, or sensed, what I interpret to be guides from another realm. Some people might call them angels. Others might consider them as indefinable quantum particles of the imagination. My perception is that they have helped, even saved, Tim on more than one occasion. My younger self censored them from the account. But I am braver now, and the world has changed. I am willing to include what I perceive to be other-worldly helpers.

An awful lot has happened in the past few years. Some of it is calling out to be included. What about the critical illness that Tim went through in Jacksonville, Florida – the one he was not expected to survive? He was 14 at the time. That's *got* to go in.

I add up the extra sections in my head. It feels as though unseen forces are nudging me gently in the right direction. Maybe this will become a published book after all.

But that's all in the future.

Just for now, let's go back in time to 1999, in Richmond, Surrey, England. My story starts with a dream.

Book One

The Miracle Child

Concerning the first three years of Timothy's life: struggles
and insights.
This account was written in 1999.

1. Shop of dreams

Last night, I dreamed I was walking along a narrow cliff path with a group of other people. I had the uncomfortable sensation of doing something I didn't want to do. Then, I just stopped. I lay down on a sloping shelf of rock and refused to go any further. Others in the party, who had been holding back from the leaders, persuaded me that I could leave the narrow path and walk directly down the hillside. So I did, and discovered it was very easy: there was nothing to be scared of.

Within minutes, I came to a promontory overlooking an airy view of an open plain. There was a shop built on the overhang: it sold clothes made of a special kind of paper. They were beautiful: like smooth, silken garments to wear close to the skin. They were even the colours of skin and parchment. I felt slightly in awe: I knew this was a special place.

The owner of the shop was a woman of my age, very friendly, and she put me at my ease. We talked for a while about the clothes, and then she directed me down, into that airy landscape which became solid and earthy beneath my feet.

I came to a building that I was reluctant to enter. Inside, I found a set of miniature figures, bluish in colour. There was a baby, lying in a manger. When I picked it up, I saw that it wasn't a conventional baby with rounded arms and legs. It was slender and long-limbed, just like our young son Timmy.

I looked closer. Entwined with the baby was a mother, wearing long robes like the Virgin Mary. And then, also entwined, I saw a little angel.

Mother, son and angel.

I felt, somehow, that I needed to breathe life into them, help them to lose that bluish colour and become pink and healthy....

I woke up this morning from that dream feeling puzzled, sad, and optimistic. A sense of beauty, truth and purpose lingered with me for hours.

Then, this afternoon, an editor at a publishing company rang me. I was half-expecting her call because our mutual friend, Tessa, had walked with her in Richmond Park and told her about Timmy, his dad Steven and me. Tessa has a knack of appearing in my life at opportune moments.

During our phone call, the editor was friendly, and keen to publish my account of Timmy's birth and first three years.

"I'd like to call it *The Miracle Child*," she said.

I wasn't sure. Would Timmy mind when he was older? But then I remembered my dream. The editor reminded me strongly of the friendly owner of the shop on the promontory. And I thought about the skin-coloured, paper clothes in her shop: they were like truthful books reflecting accurately the person inside them.

I wanted to be the sort of person who wrote truthful books – even if it hurt.

In the dream the woman had directed me downwards towards something that I felt reluctant to examine. It wasn't hard to work out why I wasn't keen. The bluish colour of the miniature figures reminded me of the day that Timmy was born. Of the moment when he had stopped breathing and turned that exact bluish shade. Despite the sad memory, the dream had felt good. And then I realised something: it's time to examine Timmy's beginnings in more detail. Doing so might help me to understand what has happened to us. It might help others in similar situations.

On one level, last night's dream seemed to be about following my own intuition and finding my own true path. In the beginning of the dream I had felt uncomfortable and eventually broke free from the prescribed route. In reality, Steven and I have felt increasingly uncomfortable with much of the medical advice we've been given, and we have learned to follow our instincts.

Timmy has benefited from our heartfelt decisions. He is

healthier and more vibrant than I think he would otherwise have been. That has to be worth telling.

Angels to look after us

There was one other element in my dream: the angel. I'm not entirely sure what this meant, but I know it has everything to do with the spiritual dimension of life. This is the part that's hardest to write about. I am not a religious person – spiritual, yes; religious, no. Nevertheless, I know that an awareness of what lies beyond the surface of life has been an influential factor in our story.

From time to time, it seems to me that I perceive another dimension, half-visible at certain moments, which seems to interface with our waking reality, and influence it benignly. This perception has not always been welcome to me. During my early career years, I managed pretty well to ignore it, and the many forms it took: quiet inner words of guidance; unusual incidents that seem to have a luminous quality; and half-glimpses of a translucent world that overlays our own. But parenting Timmy has made it impossible to ignore.

Let me give you a fairly recent example. About a year ago, there was an accident in Timmy's bedroom. It was a really silly accident that should have been avoided. I am not proud of putting my son in a dangerous position, but that is what I did.

I had just placed a steel-framed camp bed against the wall in his room. It was folded, in an upright position. It was there just for a few seconds while I repositioned another piece of furniture.

Timmy was sitting on the floor, watching my actions. Maybe he inched forwards. Certainly, he was rather closer to the frame than I had realised.

I turned around, away from the frame, away from Timmy. Without warning, the frame crashed down on to his thin legs where he was sitting on the floor. A steel frame, travelling fast… I was horrified.

Timmy said, "Oh," and looked mildly surprised.

Hardly daring to breathe, I lifted the frame from his legs.

There wasn't a scratch. Nothing. No bruise. The legs looked absolutely fine. It shouldn't have been possible, but it was. I placed the bed frame on the floor, and looked carefully for a space between the bare metal and the thin carpet. There was none: no space at all. Even taking into account a certain amount of movement from the carpet, Tim's legs should have broken the fall. By all the laws of physics, the frame should have crashed, hard, on to him. But, somehow, it didn't.

Stuff like that tends to happen around Timmy: things hard to explain, but clearly benevolent. So over time, I have moved from a state of fear, to one in which I tend to trust in the simple, invisible kindness of life.

I have also learned to listen to my dreams and they've rewarded me by becoming increasingly prophetic – like beautiful guidebooks to help me through hazardous patches that we're about to encounter.

The equation I've learnt is a simple one: if I worry and try to fix things from a state of fear, I end up messing things up.

If, on the other hand, I listen to my feelings and my intuition; if I go with opportunities that come out of the blue and somehow feel good; if I trust that things will end up well... then they generally do.

2. One year earlier

The earliest, very strange thing that I want to write about in connection with Timmy happened a year before he was born. One morning, without warning, I had a mystical experience – a spiritual vision. This changed, forever afterwards, how I thought about everything.

I wasn't, to my knowledge, ill at the time. I was in my usual state of good health. Nothing extraordinary preceded the event. I simply went to sleep. I woke up. And then it happened.

What followed does not translate easily into words. When it happened, I wasn't analysing it, or describing it in my mind. I was simply *being* the experience. I was in a state of bliss that appeared to have no beginning or end. In the account that follows, I've interwoven things I thought about afterwards, in the hope that it will make more sense to you as you read it.

A mystical experience of bliss

It's 1995, in Richmond. The sun is streaming through the bedroom window now, making patterns on the wall. It is early in the morning, and I have just opened my eyes. There is a special quality in the air: the poised, waiting quietness that comes before a town wakes up.

And in that moment, without warning, my vision alters. Although I felt no movement, all my senses are now telling me that I am no longer in Richmond. Instead, I am standing outside the back door of my grandparents' old house in Northamptonshire.

The garden here is full of flowers of every colour, and birds are singing high up in a willow tree. In the air I am aware of the scent of roses and mint, and a favourite of mine, southernwood. However, I am not actually breathing in the fragrance of these plants. I'm not even sure that I can hear the birds in the willow tree. It's more that I am absorbing some beautiful, peaceful atmosphere that consists of things like southernwood and roses.

The house – a cottage really – has thick walls made of stone. You can see that they've been whitewashed many times over, until the stones have become rounded with countless added layers of paint. The cottage is hundreds of years old. It is a place full of meaning for me, because I always felt very safe and happy here.

In my vision now, I am just entering the house; I am moving through the rooms. Curiously, I seem to have travelled back in time. The house is furnished exactly as it was when my grandparents lived there.

I go up two steps between the tiny dining room and the living room. I remember those steps well, and they bring back happy memories. We used to sit on them, my brother, sisters and I, as children, eating Grandma's fresh-made Victoria sponge cake that oozed delightfully with strawberry jam. We had big appetites from playing outdoors all day. We listened to the grown-ups chatting and we knew, without being told, that all was safe in our world.

While I am remembering that, I realise to my surprise that I am not in my body. I have no sense of my body – it's just not there. I suppose it must still be lying in bed in Richmond, but I can't locate it or get any sense of it.

This causes me no concern at all. I completely understand that spirit is my natural state. I am a floating point of consciousness.

As I move from the living room into the front room of my grandparents' old home, I become aware that I am not 'in' the house in a conventional sense. It is as if reality has shifted. This is very hard to explain. It's as if the world that we normally see is a magical type of fabric – somewhat like shot silk organza. If you look at it one way, you see the fabric. If you look at it another, you see right through the fabric and you realise that the fabric is some kind of illusion.

However, I am not simply seeing *through* the fabric. I am

actually *in* that space that is not fabric. And I can see the fabric, while also understanding that it is an illusion.

And that's only the start of it.

I have a dawning realisation that the space in which I am floating *is not empty*.

What fills the space is invisible, but I can sense it: a vast, infinite, loving presence. I am suffused in happiness to feel that presence. I feel so safe, and so loved.

I am held in that presence. I *am* that presence. I am loved and cherished by that presence. I am absolutely safe. I always have been. I always will be.

I am in bliss. I am bathing in bliss. I *am* bliss...

"This must be God," I say to myself. And with that awareness, I understand that God is everywhere, all of the time, in this deeply magical space beyond the tissue-thin illusion that we call our world.

I realise then that my previous beliefs about God are wrong. There is no judgement of any description – absolutely none. I am not, never have been and never will be a sinner. The same goes for every human on this planet. We are all loved. It's as simple as that.

When I consider all those other humans, briefly, I gain a sense of chaotic crying and unhappiness, with shafts of sunlight and order running through the whole of it.

The sunlight and order are there all the time. It feels as though people have barricaded their minds and hearts so they have forgotten virtually all the really good parts. They just get glimpses. *We* just get glimpses. I want to laugh and go up to the people and say, "Look! Wake up! Your sadness isn't real. We're all just pretending. We're just dreaming."

For some reason, during this experience all my barricades have vanished. I am entirely open to the divine sunlight. I understand that the sunshine is really just love: an infinitely accepting and nourishing love.

Slowly, I float through the downstairs rooms of my grandparents' old cottage. At every moment I feel the joy of this divine presence; I am bathing in the happiness of it. It is a feeling of indescribable happiness that has no beginning, no end. It simply continues in the most pleasing way that you can imagine.

I have no needs, no wants. I know that everything is perfect, all of the time.

Some part of me notices Grandpa's piano by a wall. It seems to shine with an internal luminescence. I realise that this luminescence has something to do with the fact that Grandpa loves, or loved, his piano.

When Grandpa played tunes for us, his eyes used to sparkle. He looked younger.

Grandpa worked hard to provide for his growing family, way back in the wartime years and beyond. His outlet – his 'me time' as we might call it today – was playing music.

Of course Grandpa had other pastimes, such as tending his vegetable garden. But that was partly an escape from the domesticity indoors. On our visits, decades later, we would often hear Grandma call him, with exasperation, into meals: "Will! Will! Where *is* he?" And he would be hidden away in the vegetable garden; or in the garage, shining his already gleaming Morris Minor.

As I observe his piano, I understand something important about Grandpa. When he played the piano he became who he truly was: not a family man; nor a working man.

When he played the piano he was simply Spirit, having fun.

I breathe in the implications of that thought. How could I have forgotten for so long? We are Spirit, and we are here to have fun.

Learning is part of the fun. We love to learn. And when we are happy, we are on track in our lives.

Happiness. Laughter. Peace. Bliss. These states of being are more real than bricks and mortar. I understand this fully now, amazed that I had ever forgotten. Love, peace and bliss are the reality behind all things.

I am pure bubbles of laughing happiness.

Slowly, I continue to float through the downstairs rooms, and on towards the staircase. I look upwards at the steep steps and the landing beyond. I remember, as a child, being tucked up in a soft bed under the eaves. My head would be full of memories of the day: walking through a field of red poppies, their papery fragrance all around me. Standing at the hawthorn hedge, patiently looking for caterpillars. And best of all, playing in the den I shared with my brother and sisters, and also with cousins.

The den was a small hut in a far corner of the garden. It had been used, a long time before, to keep pigs. Grandpa had cleaned it out and created a front door and a window. Grandma had added some old chairs, a table, a few old saucepans, plates, cups and a rusty little kettle. And Grandpa had painted a sign and nailed it up above the front door. The sign said, "Rose Cottage".

Rose Cottage was right next to a shallow, clear stream. We used to play 'houses' there, and we washed our little pots and pans in the stream when we had finished preparing our make-believe meals from leaves, berries, earth and water.

At night we would fall asleep listening to the 'swish, swish' of cars speeding by on the busy front road. The speed of the traffic and the quiet peace inside were a powerful contrast for me. They taught me that we can always choose to stop our busy lives and find peace in a quiet roadside retreat.

I am still at the bottom of the staircase. I hesitate. I'm wondering whether to go up the stairs. I would love to. But I hesitate because perhaps there are people up there, sleeping. If so, who would those people be?

The analytical questions mount up. As my left brain kicks in, the vision fades. I try to hang on to this beautiful, love-filled vision. But it's hopeless – my analytic mind has now completely taken over. The vision vanishes, and I am back in my bedroom in Richmond again.

My bedroom looks normal... but for me, *everything* has changed. I have changed. It feels as though I will never be able to look at the world the way I used to. I know the secret of what lies beyond all things. And now that I know it, I can never forget it.

A bubbling euphoria fills me up. I am bowled over by the beauty and peace and joy that can be accessed between the atoms of our world. Life is such fun. How could I ever have forgotten? I feel too euphoric to stay in bed and I jump up, dancing, as I get ready for the day.

Part of me – the analytic mind again – wonders how and why the vision happened. But I have no answer, just guesses. As far as I am aware, I am in perfect health – there is no sense that I have had a 'little death' of any sort.

It feels as though I have received special guidance, and I trust that there is a good reason why it happened to me on that day.

I have no idea – absolutely no idea – of the emotional roller coaster that lies in front of us.

3. The birth

Three years ago, when Timmy was first put into my arms, he opened his eyes and gazed straight into mine, and I was full of amazement and love, like parents often are... and I was startled too, because I felt I knew him.

We had been told by everyone except one wise woman, met at a party, that we were going to have a girl, and we had come to believe everyone, like you do. And then, on a January day, at Queen Mary's Hospital in Roehampton, our little son was born, and we said to each other: "Of course: trust him to surprise us."

I noticed that he was thin, and long-limbed – unusually so for a newborn. He was small, weighing in at just 6 lbs and 13 oz. But there was no sense of shock. He was simply, gorgeously himself.

"I don't like the sound of his breathing," said one midwife. It was true; there was a sound there, like a bubble of fluid lodged in his windpipe. But she left us anyway, in the cold birth room while the staff busied themselves elsewhere.

We were new parents, with no experience of newborns, and no experience of medical emergencies.

"What shall we call him?" I asked Steven. We hadn't even considered boys' names.

"How about Timothy?" said Steven. "It's a family name. I've always liked it."

"Timothy," I said, trying it out on my tongue. "Timmy for short."

And so, very simply, he was named.

Ninety minutes after Timmy was born, while being cradled in his father's arms in that cold birth room, our baby turned a bluish shade and stopped breathing. Steven grabbed the red emergency cord and pulled it. At that moment, we entered a nightmare world where things happen in slow motion and you are powerless to change them.

A nurse was in the room within seconds, closely followed by a paediatrician and other nameless people. Timmy was picked out of Steven's arms. He was shaken, and then given oxygen. Mercifully, he started breathing again. He was then taken immediately to the Special Care Baby Unit (SCBU), which everyone pronounced, "Skuboo", with the emphasis on the second syllable.

You don't cry when you're in the middle of a nightmare, but I'm crying now, at the memory. Actually, it's good to revisit that time, let the feelings out. No one deserves such a traumatic start to life. When we saw our little baby again, some time later, he was in an incubator, with a tube leading into his nose, a needle taped into his arm, and machines that we didn't understand, bleeping away around him.

We were told by a paediatrician that he had been given a chest X-ray, that the X-ray was inconclusive but there was a possible shadow which meant he might possibly have pneumonia, so he was on two different courses of intravenous antibiotics – hence the needle in the arm.

We accepted everything we were told. After all, we were just new, inexperienced parents. We thought the medical staff must know more than us. But later, I wished that we had been consulted. Today I don't believe Timmy had pneumonia at birth.

"I don't like the sound of his breathing," the midwife had said. Why had she left us alone all that time?

I think Timmy gradually suffocated on some amniotic fluid that hadn't been cleared. Another, stronger baby might just have coughed, and been fine. But he wasn't strong: he was small and spindly as if he hadn't grown to his full potential in the womb.

The hospital staff may well have made mistakes.

Over the past three years, Timmy has seen many doctors, and we have gone through a corresponding number of emotions concerning his devastating health issues, and the medical profession's responses to these. I have felt sadness and anger, and gratitude too.

But the truth is, what happened is history, gone. The medical staff probably did everything they knew to ensure his survival, and the fact that he is here today is by far and away the most important thing.

I believe that every medical person we've encountered, then or since, has always had good intentions, even though, over time, I have come to believe they are often misguided.

As we stood over our son in his incubator, the paediatrician who was explaining everything said to us, "We'll probably need to do a lumbar puncture." And that shook me out of the nightmare, just enough to say, "Why?"

The doctor looked surprised, and said that perhaps it wouldn't be necessary, and the suggestion didn't come up again.

It was going to be many months before we felt more in control of the situation. But that little word "Why?" was the first tiny starting point. We'd saved our son from an unnecessary and painful test, and that felt good.

That evening, Steven went home, I went to the maternity ward, and Timmy was left in SCBU. Leaving him there felt like a continuation of the nightmare. Like many parents before me I thought, "It's not supposed to be like this."

In the maternity ward I dreamed vividly that the faces of countless tiny newborn babies were facing me, their little mouths open like the mouths of baby birds. They wanted food: I could hear the words, "Feed me, feed me."

It felt as though they were asking for nourishment in its fullest sense. They were silently asking me to look after them. And all the faces looked the same: it was Timmy's face, seen many times over, as if in a distorting mirror – as if holographically spread across immense space.

I woke with an immense feeling of pressure and responsibility. It felt as though there was so much to do, and I didn't know how to do it.

Three years later, I can still feel that pressure, like a gossamer weight composed of countless wishes. Who can say for sure what a dream means? However, I favour three possible interpretations.

The first interpretation: the dream was about Timmy. It showed my perception that Timmy was, somehow, not fully in his body. It felt almost as though he was somehow fragmentary in this physical plane. He was occupying *all* of space, not just the narrow physical frame which was supposed to be his earthly vessel.

The second interpretation: the dream was about children with special needs, or disabilities. I was going to become busy writing for parents of children with cognitive and physical disabilities. I felt the dream babies were telling me there was an overwhelming need for this. Maybe I saw it like that because I like to communicate – it is my therapy, my way of working out what I actually think about things. And in healing myself this way, it can also happen that I offer something to others in a similar situation.

The third interpretation: the dream was about me. Dream analysts, from Carl Jung to the present day, view everything and everyone in a dream as a symbolic reflection of the dreamer. Babies may symbolise the undeveloped aspects, or even projects, of the dreamer. These projects may require care, attention and nourishment to come to fruition.

Which interpretation do I choose? Today, I accept all three. They work together for me, on different levels.

Until recently, though, I found the second explanation easiest to deal with – because it provided me with an outlet I desperately needed.

I've written ever since I can remember. As an adult, I've written countless articles and a couple of books which all aimed to help people find their optimum career, relationship... their optimum life.

In my writing, I've always tended towards a positive, self-empowering, inspiring outlook.

If there's any area that needs this kind of positive outlook, it's the area of children's disabilities.

As I was just beginning to find out, when your child has serious health problems and/or developmental delays, you enter a dreary world of medical tests, doom-laden predictions and painful treatments.

Over time, you will spend many hours in unappealing waiting rooms, decorated with negative posters showing photos of harmful bacteria and other toxic images.

You won't know how long you'll be waiting for, but eventually, you will be summoned into the presence of a doctor. This doctor will, for the purest of all possible reasons, leave you tearful and without hope.

Optimism, self-esteem, laughter and everyday normality will all vanish from your life for long periods.

During this time, many experts will give you advice about your child and your life. All of them will have trained for years to collect unpronounceable sets of capital letters that they will proudly place after their names on the dreary hospital correspondence they send you. And you will have no qualifications to speak of: you are just a parent, just a human being!

In the face of all this you will probably, at least at the beginning, stifle your own intuitive parental feelings in favour of their textbook instructions. After all, 'doctors know best'. But something won't feel right, and you will be left feeling miserable and uncomfortable.

We weren't aware of any of this at the beginning. Like countless parents before us, we were completely unprepared for the job. All we had was a little baby in SCBU, and a perplexing dream to guide us.

Today, I would give my baby boy healing. By this, I mean that I would reach a state of inner calm; gain a peaceful sense of Tim and myself as manifestations of the infinite; and visualise healing light from the universal energy field entering his body and his own energy field, helping him in myriad ways.

I wish I'd known that then.

But our babies are our best teachers. They can teach us how to become parents, if we will only listen to them.

After 48 hours of observation with no further incident, Timmy was allowed to join me in the maternity ward. That night, it seemed as though he came back from his own nightmare, one that had kept him quiet and inert in SCBU. He was suddenly more wriggly and lively.

First, I breastfed him, and then I gave him a top-up bottle of formula milk. The hospital recommended top-up bottles and supplied them liberally. Today, I would refuse them outright. Today, I know that breast milk supplies adjust naturally to meet demand. Giving a baby formula milk gets in the way of that process.

But the hospital was erring on the side of caution. "When in doubt, intervene," might have been their unwritten motto.

After the feed, I tried to put Timmy in his little plastic cot by my hospital bed, just as all the other mothers had done with their babies. But Timmy cried and cried until I lay him down over my chest. And then he fell instantly asleep.

"He knows what he wants," I thought. Feeling as reassured by his little presence as he felt by mine, I closed my eyes and slept.

4. The first year

Every parent is terrified of cot death. Our son had already stopped breathing once; we had reason to be scared. In the hospital I asked a midwife whether she thought we should get a breathing monitor for Timmy's cot at home. She looked at me, smiled a very sweet smile and said, "Look to the baby, not to machines."

Her feeling was that parents tune into their babies, and that machines can get in the way of that process. Steven and I both felt her words made sense. I am truly grateful for her brave advice, because it relieved us from months of panicking over false alarms. Timmy did not stop breathing again, and showed no signs of doing so.

At four weeks he started smiling; by six weeks his smiles were definite and frequent. Later we learned that this is generally considered a good sign, as babies with delays are often slow to smile – sometimes very slow.

But we soon began to realise that everything was not all right. At around three months we noticed that his head wasn't growing as quickly as the rest of him. The difference was subtle at first, but over the first year it became more obvious. At first he gained weight well, but that began to slow too.

Other, worrying signs began to appear. He didn't start grasping things as quickly as his peers. And, puzzlingly, his middle fingers couldn't straighten.

There were other odd things. He tended to lie with his head facing left. He used his legs more than his hands. His arms were very sensitive: he would cry if you raised them above his head. He would squint in the bright light outdoors. He was slow to roll over. His head control was poor. There was no sign of him sitting up, let alone crawling.

He was also very volatile. We discovered early on that Timmy at home and Timmy in the wider world were two quite different people.

Timmy at home

With us, he was just lovely. He was responsive to cuddles. He showed a sense of humour at a surprisingly early age. He laughed at little mishaps and surprises. If you pretended to fall over a toy, for example, he would find it hilarious, laughing in a characteristic silent way, his whole face creased up, his eyes sparkling.

He was extremely watchful: he appeared to be observing everything. He avoided eye contact, although he did look at us, his parents, at least some of the time. Occasionally at night, when the light was dim, he would gaze endlessly into my eyes. These were wonderful moments.

He loved books from early on: looking at the images any which way; being read to.

He was also fascinated by sunlight and shadows. He would move a hand and watch the shadow moving too, then turn his head to look for the source of the light.

Sometimes he would get upset when the normal laws of physics weren't observed. One time, for example, he was watching *Teletubbies* on TV. Usually he enjoyed this programme. He particularly liked watching the Teletubbies glide down the slide that deposited them into the centre of their grassy home.

But on this occasion the law of gravity was defied, and the Teletubbies slid *up* their slide instead of down. Timmy cried out, evidently disturbed by this impossibility.

Timmy in the wider world

Outside our home, he was a different child. He gazed nowhere in particular. He cried easily. He appeared spaced out and overwhelmed. Eye contact all but disappeared. In places with lots of echoes – such as houses and restaurants with bare floorboards – he would cry endlessly and we would have to take him home early.

I suspected that he had synaesthesia – that his senses were jumbled up in places. I thought this because he seemed to react to sounds as though he could *see* them.

Often, when he heard music or many voices, his eyes would move watchfully over empty space, as though he was, perhaps, seeing patterns of light and colour.

When this happened, he would smile and coo, as though what he saw was pleasing. At times it looked just as if he could see an invisible person, someone he knew and loved. "He's talking to his guardian angel," I once told an aunt of Steven's at a family wedding.

Timmy didn't turn his head to the direction of sound, and this was one of the things that his health visitor and doctors picked up on. They thought he might be deaf. We knew he wasn't, but we had to jump through the hoops. He had to sit through a succession of hearing tests, all of which he failed. One day a wise consultant said, "I'm sure he can hear, so I'm going to discharge him, and if you have any worries, just come back to me."

The torture of testing

Consultants. Perhaps I'd better talk about them. It's time I admitted they are not my favourite subject. We have met some wonderful individuals. But we have also met a fair number who seem to get the wrong end of the stick. It's as if we speak completely different languages.

We've never met a consultant who saw Timmy as we see him. I suppose they come to the problem very differently. They are trained to identify anomalies – deviations from the norm. When they find any deviations, they test in a variety of ways to try to find the cause.

But if, like Timmy, a child does not fit into an easily identified syndrome, the testing continues until the parents say, "Enough!"

The testing was painful and upsetting for Timmy and I loathed my role of putting him into a position of suffering in this way. And it *was* my role, as I was the main carer. Sometimes Steven was present, especially for the bigger tests. But a lot of the time it was just Timmy and me.

There were, it almost goes without saying, many blood tests. It's hard to find a vein in a small baby's arm, hand or foot, so there was often trauma, even terror.

There was a particularly horrible investigation that involved injecting a radioactive substance into Timmy's urethra and then seeing how it travelled through his urinary system. The substance was injected through his penis. He was spread-eagled on the table, resisting furiously, screaming in pain and fear. An old friend accompanied me for that one and he was visibly shaken, as was I.

Timmy had to be held down, and he was screaming and screaming. TV screens documented the radioactive chemical's journey through his body. The old friend who accompanied me was completely horrified. He thought Steven should have been there, but bit the words back. "Well, he's not here, and that's all there is to say," was his restrained verdict. I was grateful to him for his support.

That particular test was done because scans showed that Timmy had a horseshoe kidney, where the two kidneys had fused together in the womb. Doctors explained there can be a risk of reflux, so that's what they were trying to discover.

Timmy had never shown any symptoms, however. And the test results, thankfully, were negative.

The testing continued relentlessly. At around five months, Timmy had an overnight stay at the Royal Brompton Hospital for an endoscopy. Steven was with us that time. A camera was to be put down Timmy's throat and into his upper air passages. The test was for a suspected floppy larynx, which we didn't believe he had.

Before the procedure, Timmy was given a general anaesthetic, but he strongly resisted going under.

"We had to give him quite a bit more than the usual dose," admitted the anaesthetist afterwards. "Nearly double in fact."

Steven and I stared anxiously at our heavily drugged son. His breathing was so laboured – we'd never heard it so bad.

"Does he usually breathe like that?" asked the anaesthetist. "You've heard him breathe like that before, I expect?"

"Not until we came here," said Steven.

It upset both Steven and me that the medical testing, yet again, seemed to be doing more harm than good.

A couple of months later, Timmy was admitted to Queen Mary's Hospital in Roehampton. There, a nasogastric tube was inserted through one of his nostrils and down into his oesophagus. There was a pH probe on the end, to measure whether acid was leaving his stomach and going up into the oesophagus.

The pH probe was the test that made me most angry and upset. I was sure that he didn't suffer from reflux, as it's called, and yet I wasn't confident enough to refuse the test. We also didn't feel the test was explained in any detail in advance.

"We'd better do a pH probe," said the paediatrician, and that was more or less that.

I would love it if doctors tried some of the techniques they prescribe for their patients – just to see what they feel like.

During the two days of the reflux test, Timmy kept pulling the nasogastric tube out and it had to be forced down again, through his nose, into his stomach. I had to hold him down while this was being done, like a warder restraining a prisoner who is being force-fed. This was so upsetting. It seemed to me that I should be stopping people from hurting Timmy, and instead I was helping them.

To prevent him from pulling the tube out, his little hands were bandaged up, but he managed to pull it out one more time anyway. By that stage the test was nearly over, so they just gave up.

The results for each and every test were either negative, or inconclusive.

Some of the most absurd testing simply involved observing Timmy for anomalies.

"His ears seem unusually low," said one doctor. "They're in the normal place," decided several others.

"One big toe is longer than the other," said another doctor.

"He's just Timmy; we all come in different shapes and sizes," I wanted to say, but I didn't. I also politely refrained from asking if the doctor's own big toes were a perfect match.

I didn't say these things because I was not used to questioning people in authority. I was aware, as every parent quickly becomes aware, that medical staff supposedly do things in a particular, 'scientific' way. Of course many of the methods used are not scientific, but we're not supposed to mention that, or even notice.

Steven and I also had the impression that our own observations about Timmy were ignored. It was as if the doctors were going through a 'tick the box' questionnaire.

For example, when Timmy was undergoing hearing tests I said, "I'm sure he can hear perfectly well, it's just that he has problems processing what he hears – and I think he might have synaesthesia because he appears to watch sound."

The consultant raised her eyebrows briefly, *but then completely ignored my words*. The only way I could explain this strange indifference to parental observation was this: there was no box on her questionnaire for synaesthesia, so it didn't exist.

One day, Timmy was breathing heavily and a rather bossy young doctor commented on it. She started writing a note about it.

"When does he make that noise, Mum?" she asked, pen poised, waiting for my answer. I was still not used to being called "Mum" by medics at that time, and I didn't like it.

"When he's concentrating," I answered, truthfully.

Her pen lowered. "I can't write that down!"

"Why not?"

"It's not... precise enough."

"But it's true."

In the end she gave up.

Nearly every time we saw a consultant, they scared and upset me. That in itself had a negative effect on Timmy. The psychology of dealing tactfully with worried parents is not, it would appear, one of the things that doctors learn – but really it should be.

Some of the consultants were likeable, and rather distinguished in an academic sort of way. They might have been fun to meet at a dinner party or some other social event.

One or two appeared power-mad within the hospital hierarchy. Perhaps this is unfair, but I actually got the impression they enjoyed putting young children and parents through unnecessary tests.

One consultant, the nurses confessed to us, actually went by the nickname of Cruella de Vil among the staff.

And we also came across the occasional consultant who was clearly too overworked and overstressed to make any sensible decisions at all.

Virtually all the consultants were very careful not to give us any false hopes, which meant they gave no hope at all. Through the holistic literature that I was beginning to read, I learned there was a name for this approach: the 'nocebo response'. This term was coined in the 1960s. Nowadays it's generally called the nocebo effect.

The nocebo effect can operate like a witch doctor's curse. When we receive a poor prognosis from a person we respect, we have a strong tendency to believe it even if it isn't true. Our body acts as if it is true, and in this way it can become a self-fulfilling prophecy.

The nocebo effect did have an impact on me. After every

appointment I felt more negative, more fearful and more powerless. I also felt angry that I was letting myself be affected in this way. I could see what was happening. I just couldn't work out how to stop it. I knew my despondency was bad for Timmy. But I still couldn't stop it.

Looking back on those early months, I can see more clearly now the psychological harm the whole process caused the three of us. I can see how it coloured our parenting of Timmy. It took away some of the spontaneity of loving a little child, and replaced it with an anxious surveillance. It took away a lot of the pride I had in my son, and replaced this with sadness and guilt.

Steven and I also drifted apart at this time. "I'm not ready for this," he said at one point.

"Who is?" I wondered.

Steven became an occasional presence in the house, and absent from more hospital appointments. For long periods, I was effectively a single parent. I was very upset about that, but my priority was Timmy, whom I adored.

I felt I must have done something wrong for him to be the way he was. I went through waves and waves of guilt. I also felt that by not knowing what to do for the best now, I was letting my son down all over again.

Meanwhile, the tests results continued to show nothing. Blood, urine, sweat and X-rays... there was still no diagnosis. There was no neat label to explain his condition.

Through a writer's eyes

Steven and I were both earning our living as writers and editors, and that gave us a particular perspective. Steven, who has a clear, analytical mind, was particularly good at noticing when doctors expressed opinions masquerading as facts. Sometimes I envied him, because he occupied a world of facts and certainty more completely than me.

My mind worked in a different, more intuitive way, in which

conflicting realities seemed to coexist. So I would, for example, see and hear a doctor talking, but look beyond the surface words, into the origins of how they came to think and express themselves that way.

It may be helpful to explain how I came to think in this multilayered manner.

At the time I was working as a freelance writer for a range of magazines and the occasional newspaper. But more than that, I had a love of story that went back as far as my earliest reading days. As a child, I was a compulsive reader. When I was deep in a book, I resented interruptions. I wanted to continue in that heady space where the author's imagination interfaced with my own.

English was my favourite subject at school, by a long way. Because my family moved around a lot, my older sister and I went to a state boarding school in the Norfolk countryside. The land was flat all around. The skies provided much of the magic. I would gaze up at the stars at night, and envisage a kind, guiding consciousness gazing back at me.

In those days, fewer school leavers went on to further education, the way they do today. There weren't nearly so many universities. However, when I was in the Sixth Form a new teacher decided that some of the brightest students should try for the University of Cambridge. He took a group of us on a tour to meet a few admissions tutors.

The first college we saw was Trinity, and I fell in love with it. There was something about those strings of mellow-stoned rooms around peaceful courtyards that was hugely appealing. It was the atmosphere of learning – of people following their own heartfelt interests – that drew me. I also thought the location was delightful. In front of the college was an interesting and quirky town to explore. Behind the college lay the green spaces of nature with the River Cam running through it all. Trinity looked like the perfect place for learning and imagination to flourish.

I was lucky enough to be accepted to read English. I arrived as a very unconfident 18 year old. I felt inferior to the worldly, privately-educated students who in many cases had gained experience abroad during a gap year. But gradually, I found my way.

For three years, my only task was to study literature. I learned to look for the deepest layers of meaning in a text. I became impatient with published critical interpretations. I didn't want 'middle men' telling me what the author meant. I wanted to connect directly with the author, through their written words. "You have to go back to the source," I would say, both to myself and to anyone who listened. "Go directly to the source."

That was my mantra and it still rings true for me today.

Without realising it, during that period I also developed a practical philosophy for life that broadly came down to three words.

"Life is story."

It seemed to me that each human being lives his or her own story from birth to death, and maybe beyond. Within each life story there are many chapters. These chapters may sometimes appear to be short stories in their own right, but they are always related to the whole. Each of us has our own big theme to grapple with. The themes are concepts like forgiveness, understanding, empathy, trust, compassion and balance. Beyond these, the giant theme that runs through every life story is unconditional love – and fear, its antithesis.

I was aware that stories, like music, have certain rules that make them so. Without the rules there would be cacophony, or chaos. In a story there needs to be a beginning, a middle and an end. There has to be a character, or characters. There has to be some kind of event, often difficult, hopefully transformative, through which the central character lives and changes for the better. There has to be motivation. There has to be a sequence that makes sense: cause must lead to effect.

After I left Cambridge and went to London to work, I entered a very different world of commercial writing, mainly for glossy consumer magazines. There, I discovered a schism in me. I could no longer read, or write, authentically. I had to subedit and write what the publishers believed would sell. There was always a compromise. I never became fully comfortable with that compromise, but I did continue to learn about human nature, and the stories, and lies, we tell ourselves.

I also learned to spot when someone lies.

This is how it happens. Each of us lives our story. The story flows, in natural sequence. However, if someone lies, his or her story pauses. It stops, momentarily. There is a jarring sensation as the story stops – it's subtle, but clearly present if you know what you are looking for. And then, the story continues a little differently.

Just look for the *non sequitur*. Look for a pause. Look for an answer that is different to the question that was asked. That's where you'll find the boarded-up parts of the psyche, within which the shadow self dwells.

I learned something else which struck me as a revelation: most people are not aware when they are lying. It is an unconscious process. People lie when they cannot face the truth. People lie many times over, all through their lives, when they cannot face certain fundamental truths. These truths aren't 'out there'. They are within a person's own psyche.

So therefore, I reasoned, to be a good, authentic storyteller we must work on our own hidden areas. We must uncover our own shadow self. We must embrace that which we find difficult within ourselves.

And now, as a new mother, I was silently applying those same principles to Timmy's doctors.

I understood that each doctor we met had worked really hard to become qualified. They were high achievers – perfectionists.

I could understand perfectionism. I had big doses of it myself.

But there's something any perfectionist needs to ask him or herself, sooner or later. In a roundabout way I have my well-meaning father, who always wanted the best for me, to thank for the following insight.

Let's say I had got 93% in a school exam. My dad would ask, "What happened to the other 7%?"

It used to drive me crazy. I thought we should celebrate the high result I had achieved, instead of lamenting the dropped marks. But I would try harder the next time, and achieve a little bit more. And so I became a high achiever.

On a deeper level, my father's question had an altogether different answer. On a deeper level, the proportion of me that had failed – the 7% – did go somewhere. It went to the unchartered recesses of my shadow self. I disowned the part of me that didn't or couldn't make the grade. But it was real and couldn't physically vanish. So instead it lay hidden deep within me, until such a time as I would see it reflected in my outer world.

And then I gave birth to a son who exemplified that 7%. He couldn't pass any tests. He couldn't reach any developmental milestones. He was, by the standards of any Schools Examining Board, an absolute failure. And I adored him. Learning to love and accept Timmy wasn't difficult. He was full of unconditional love. But learning to love and accept him created a major change in *me*, because it gave me permission to love that hidden aspect of me – the 7% that failed, that was less than perfect.

Those high-achieving doctors also had their less-than-perfect shadow selves. But I wondered how aware any of them were of this fundamental fact. If they were unaware, the children with disabilities they treated were carrying a heavy burden. The unaware doctors could project all their imperfections on to the children, and remain resolutely superior. Not in a nasty way, of course. But still....

Even worse, on a deeper level there would be no real impetus to change the status quo – to bring about genuine healing. The perfectionist needs failures around them, in order to measure their own success.

Does this sound unkind? I don't mean to be. I'm fully aware that countless lives have been saved in hospitals, including – as we shall see – my son's.

But I do wonder whether medical students study their *own* psyches sufficiently in medical schools. I suspect there's not much time for it, but there should be, because it would create better, and happier, doctors.

Sometimes I would notice that a particular medic loved the power. Perhaps they enjoyed saying things with little risk of being challenged. Perhaps deep down they were insecure, and this is how it manifested.

The younger doctors might, one would hope, bring fresh thinking to the profession. But conservatism was king.

I noticed how the younger doctors had traded their individuality for the security of group thinking. I could see how very proud they were to belong to that group.

I could understand the pride, up to a point. Medics work hard for many years to gain their qualifications. They aren't likely to question the system as soon as they're fully qualified members, especially since they are still low down in the hierarchy, and dependent on the good will of their seniors.

But group thinking can be dangerous. In a group, individual responsibility may give way to group responsibility. Poor decisions can be made in specific cases because a senior member has created a general rule that is supposed to apply to all. Even if a junior member secretly believes the senior member is wrong, the boss is still obeyed.

Alongside poor specific decisions, there can be arrogance and a misguided feeling of superiority. All these factors create a 'glass wall' between medics and their patients. The glass wall prevents the medics feeling empathy, or indeed *any* emotional connection, with the patients.

What it really means to be a patient

The term 'patient' is most revealing.

Words matter. I love to look at their original meanings.

Here is a dictionary definition of the word 'patient':

Patient: from the Latin, 'pati', meaning 'to suffer, to endure'. Enduring without complaint. Capable of accepting delay with equanimity.

Maybe that explains all the tortuous waiting times built into the British health care system! We wait for appointments. When we do reach the hospital, we can spend hours on end in depressing waiting rooms.

There is nothing in the word 'patient' to suggest wellness, or the process of getting better. It's all about waiting, and enduring.

If you want to get better, get impatient.

A questionnaire for medics

I believe that paediatric doctors do need to ask themselves how empathetic they are towards their young patients.

Here are three good questions any paediatric physician might consider:

- What does it feel like to be a child undergoing tests, week after week?
- Would it ultimately be better for that child to have fewer tests and a happier lifestyle?
- If I, the paediatrician, dared to give the family hope, would that improve the child's chances of thriving?

And here is a deeper question that every medic should ask:

- How can I know myself better?

Even if the experts are attempting to act for the best – and I am sure the overwhelming majority are doing just that – the reality is they do not and should not hold the power.

The power for the child's well-being should be with the child. If the child can't speak for him or herself, the power should be with the parents, or those who fulfil the role of loving the child.

Consultants are called consultants because that is exactly what they are supposed to be. We consult them in their particular area of expertise – and then we make up our own mind, having considered their professional opinion.

During Timmy's first year I encountered many other parents of disabled children and I began to realise that parents often do not have the full facts. We feel disenfranchised from a system that keeps most of the knowledge to itself and feeds its patients a blend of dumbed-down leaflets and prescriptions with unduly complex names. These names derive from Latin yet would *never* have been spoken by any self-respecting citizen of ancient Rome.

If you are alive on this planet, you are normal

I was beginning to wonder why the more extreme variations of a young human body should be seen as 'medical' anyway. Was it possible, I wondered, that at times we 'medicalise' our children unnecessarily?

I was beginning to understand that the way disabled children are viewed by the wider world – as though there is something wrong with them – is in itself wrong.

It seemed to me that we should be trying to see the world through the children's eyes. We should be learning from them, and helping them to grow up as happy, healthy *normal* people with their own particular blend of strengths and weaknesses.

You noticed I used the word *"normal"*?

This is what I believe. If you are alive on this planet, you are normal. No exceptions. We are not identical robots off some biological assembly line. Variations in human beings are *normal*.

From my experience with Timmy, and from meetings with other disabled children, I was beginning to feel that our children are often brighter than doctors suppose. This was an eye-opener for me. Before I had Timmy, I had always assumed that a child or adult with learning difficulties is, in some way, 'sub-intelligent' – less intelligent than the rest of us.

But after I had Timmy, I realised that while he couldn't pass standard developmental tests, he was observant, with a keen sense of humour, and a good grasp of how the physical world behaved. He also appeared hyper-aware in certain respects. For example, my friend Julie noticed that if I walked out of her living room while Timmy was sleeping, he would invariably wake up and cry out for me. "How does he know you're leaving?" she would marvel.

The problem was not that he was vegetable in his intelligence. The problem was that some aspects of his nervous system, including his sensory system, didn't seem to work conventionally. There may have been pain and discomfort associated with this, but that wasn't the sort of question any medical person asked.

I wasn't sure why these basic, core issues weren't being addressed.

Insight into Timmy's mind

You and I may not know what it feels like to have our sensory processing jumbled up. But this is how I think it may be for my son....

Just imagine that you're feeling ill and tired, and all you want to do is rest and recover, but you keep having to go to white, harshly-lit doctors' rooms and do tests. You don't understand what the tests are for. You know from previous experience that you may endure physical pain.

You know that the adult carer with you – your mother – is upset but trying not to show it. But, being hypersensitive, you can pick up her distress as clearly as if she is shouting. Actually, to you, her silent distress is a loud, audible cry.

You also pick up the emotions of the white-coated adults in the room with you. There's one who is thinking, loudly and angrily, about some aspect of her private life that has nothing to do with you, but she has brought the emotion with her anyway. It's a loud emotion, and it hurts you. There's another who has written you off. He thinks you're thin and misshapen. He's fairly certain you won't last through childhood, but he's going through the motions of trying to help you.

Thankfully, there's another who is radiating kindness and it soothes you. But unfortunately, there's a bright light all along the ceiling and it pulses erratically and noisily, many times a second. It makes you feel dizzy and sick, which mixes up with your fear and tiredness so you feel simply terrible. The adults don't seem to notice the effect but it's hurting you.

You also don't like the strange, antiseptic smell in the room. It's the opposite of homely. You just want to go home, away from all these horrible sensations.

In those circumstances, would you bloom... or would you avoid everyone's eyes and simply shriek?

Supportive family and friends

In between appointments, home was a welcome relief. There was such a contrast between the depressing hospital atmosphere, and the comfort of home. The little house we lived in – in Albany Passage, Richmond – always seemed like a sanctuary. There was kindness built into the walls. We had kind neighbours and good local friends. We had one family member close by – a brother of Steven's. He and his wife were supportive in helpful, practical ways.

My parents lived a hundred miles away in Wiltshire, and Steven's parents were further away, in the north of England, so we didn't see as much of them as we would have liked, but they still managed to help enormously in terms of supportive comments. Every one of our four parents has been an immense help, and we will always be hugely grateful to them.

Some of their worry was occasionally difficult to deal with. Steven's mother was always warm-hearted and caring, and quick to travel to us to give whatever support was required. However, things did become strained between the two of us for a little while. She didn't understand the value of breastfeeding – it was simply outside her experience. She thought Timmy would thrive if we would only feed him formula milk with a bit of rusk dissolved in it. In fact, his growth charts at that time showed that he put on the most weight during the short period when he was solely breastfed. But I struggled with the unspoken pressure to 'feed him up', and I'm sure she must have struggled with my parenting approach that would have seemed so different to hers.

I would like to say this is not a criticism of her, or the many parents who bottle-feed their babies. Hopefully, we each get to choose the path that is best for our particular circumstances.

For me, breastfeeding was the obvious choice, because that was the way I had been brought up. My mother had breastfed each of her four babies. This skill had never been lost in my maternal line. Both my parents grew up in families who loved nature. To this day, my parents grow many of their own fruit and vegetables. They believe in the natural goodness of nature, and they are healthier than many of their generation.

My parents were also very good at coming up with reasons why Timmy would be all right.

They decided, for example, that Timmy looked just like my great-grandpa. William Russell-Davis had been a very sickly baby. He had not been expected to last the year. But William confounded the doctors. In fact, he outlived all of them. He died eventually at the ripe old age of 103.

"Grandpa was stubborn," my mother said, "very stubborn."

They thought Timmy had inherited that determined streak, and so did I.

The very first example of Timmy's stubbornness had actually come when I was just 10 weeks' pregnant. It was an early intimation that all was not right. Over a period of days, I experienced excruciating pain, followed by copious bleeding as if a tap had been turned on. I had felt very emotional during that time, awash in a tidal surge of saltwater tears. I was so sad at the thought of losing my baby.

I remember Tessa turned up on the most painful day, bearing ingredients for a healthy lunch. I hardly felt like eating, but I truly appreciated her support.

Our baby, amazingly, hung on. And eventually he was born, small but punctual, on his due date.

I was also blessed with an extremely good group of friends whom I'd met at my NHS antenatal classes. Long after our classes had finished, we just kept on meeting, and we still do to this day. At the same time I met and became good friends with other local mothers, so I've always felt surrounded by friendship.

There was a phase though, during the first summer, when I began to find excuses not to meet up with my friends.

It was around the time that their babies began to sit up. Week after week, I'd see the other babies moving effortlessly through their milestones. They would sit up, hold on to rattles and make the first pre-crawl moves. Timmy was doing none of these things, although he enjoyed lolling around and watching.

Also, I couldn't help but notice how different Timmy looked from them. They were all round and chubby, while Timmy stayed comparatively long-limbed and spindly.

I found the differences upsetting, and didn't know how to deal with them. Yet I still enjoyed meeting up. My friends and I still seemed to have a lot in common, and there was always plenty to talk about.

Around the same time, the community paediatrician was steering me gently towards a local special needs social group.

I took Timmy along a couple of times, to see what it was like. It didn't seem like my kind of thing. There were health professionals there to oversee us, so we couldn't truly relax. It seemed forced somehow. Timmy didn't enjoy it either.

Meanwhile, Carolyn or Louise or one of my other friends from the antenatal group would be on the phone, asking how I was, having a natter, offering a lift to the next get-together... just being normal. And I liked that. So I carried on meeting them. We talked a bit about Timmy's slowness, and the tests, but it wasn't a big thing, it was just one of the many subjects we talked about. That suited me.

Double vision

It felt as though I was seeing life through two different lenses at the same time.

On the one hand, Timmy was showing serious delays and just not thriving. We were enduring a puzzlement of paediatricians who were doing tests, saying horrible things, making Timmy and me cry (though I generally saved my tears for home).

On the other hand, I was a new mother who felt full of love and pride for her baby. I'd push him in his pram or carry him in his sling around Richmond, and I never, ever felt that anyone looked at him oddly. Absolutely the contrary: people came up to us, fussed over him and said he was sweet, cute, and beautiful.

"Oh, if only I had my camera. This moment will never happen again," cried one woman, gazing adoringly into his blue eyes. Timmy was sitting forwards-facing in a baby sling on that occasion, and he did look particularly cute like that.

"Ooh, those eyelashes, you could sweep the road with them," sighed another lady. It's true, he did have very long and luxuriant eyelashes.

As with all babies, wherever we went there'd be people nearby dissolving into smiles at the sight of him. (Today, aged three, he still has this effect. Just this morning I took him on a bus to my friend Julie's house in Twickenham for the group's weekly get-together. Fellow passengers all around were smiling at him. One started a little game of 'Where's my ticket?' with him. Timmy's face was creased up with laughter.)

Occasionally, someone would come up to us and say, "Your son has a really unusual face; he is beautiful."

But I could never become *too* proud and happy about my baby, because the medical scrutiny continued relentlessly.

The medics also thought he was unusual. But the way they said it was not flattering. Several said that they'd never met anyone like him before.

It would have satisfied their tidy minds if they could have tucked him into a syndrome, but which one? Nothing seemed to fit. In the middle of their note taking they'd look up and see Timmy's eyes watchfully on them and they'd hesitate, confused.

A particularly low point came when Timmy's consultant said he might have a chromosomal or genetic abnormality. There's something about these words that can sound ugly. They touched a nerve.

I was just beginning to understand that inclusion mattered a lot to me. I was developing the view that we are all special, all equal, and each of us is unique. With this dawning awareness came the acceptance that each of us has a different genetic code, and that's fine – we are meant to be diverse.

But the medical probing seemed to carry a different vibration. I was feeling sensitive about this – perhaps overly so. It seemed to me that there was an implication that if your code didn't match up, you didn't belong in the club. The club was for normal people. If your genetic code didn't match up, you weren't normal. You were abnormal.

At home on the morning of the chromosomal test I gazed at my baby, wondering how his blueprint might be different from mine and other people's. I was aware of a voice somewhere deep inside me. The voice was protesting vigorously.

"Timmy is not 'different', at least, not in a bad way," said the voice – my voice. "He is my child. He is totally lovable and accepted by me. He is as close to me as any human ever could be."

And then we caught the bus along the Sheen Road to Queen Mary's Hospital. We had to wait. I carried Timmy into the hospital garden, and there, I started crying. I really did feel low about the whole thing. However, Sarah, one of the mothers from my antenatal group, found me there and was very comforting. Her son was in for a minor operation. That made me realise that Timmy and I were not completely the odd ones out.

"This one is special."

After the chromosome test there was an inevitable wait for the results. During this period, I felt a strong need for some 'sanctuary' time, away from medical appointments.

I took Timmy to visit my family in Wiltshire. Ever since my parents moved there, just after I left Cambridge, I have always loved this part of England. It's quiet and peaceful. Plants and perhaps people grow well there. Wiltshire contains rolling chalk downs, and an abundance of atmospheric, prehistoric sites. My parents lived not far from the sacred stone circle of Avebury, and mysterious Silbury Hill.

On the road from London, just after Avebury, you drive through a gap in trees. It's always felt like a gateway to me. Once I was through that gateway, I could relax.

On this particular trip I went to the local medieval village of Lacock with my older sister. Lacock – pronounced 'Laycock' – has been used in countless films, including Jane Austen's *Pride and Prejudice*, and *Harry Potter* movies. It's a beautiful and rather magical place, dating back to a time when science and mythology could exist comfortably on the same map.

We were in a tea garden, when a slender, elderly, silver-haired lady came up to us. She made a fuss of Timmy. Then she looked at me, with clear blue eyes.

"This one is special," she said. "You'll need to take extra care of this one."

And she explained that she used to be a children's nurse.

After she left, my sister and I gazed at each other: a 'what was all that about!' sort of look. The silver-haired lady had appeared as if from nowhere and then disappeared so quickly after she had delivered her message.

Unfortunately, it wasn't a message I had asked for, and it wasn't a welcome message. Did she think I was unaware? Did she think it was her business to tell me the obvious?

I realised then that I was angry with the silver-haired lady.

I was angry that she had courteously spelt out that Timmy had serious health issues.

And I was angry that she was right.

Dreaming of recompression

Soon after this, I had a curious dream – the sort of dream that feels real, albeit on a different level to normal waking life.

I was walking into a large room. It was a light, featureless space. I saw no detail whatsoever, except for the following: in the middle of the room there was a platform, like the sort of table a patient might lie on in an operation. Timmy was lying on the table. He didn't seem worried, or upset. He appeared to be sound asleep.

Around him were perhaps five or six tall figures. Again, they had no particular features. They were simply tall and elongated. It seemed to me that light emanated from them. In my mind, I called them "people of light".

The closest one turned to me, and moved slightly towards me in a welcoming way. There was no sense of legs moving to and fro; it seemed more as if the figure were gliding. I wasn't sure whether it was male or female. It was really just an elongated being of light.

I wasn't afraid, but I did want to know what was happening. I wanted to be sure that Timmy was safe.

The being of light spoke to me, but not with lips. It was as if the words arrived fully formed in my mind.

"We are recompressing him."

The energy behind the words seemed... awesome. There was a sense of kindness and love. There was also the impression that these beings had capabilities far beyond anything I knew of. I felt reassured, and happy. I had the sudden realisation that we were not alone in this difficult situation. We were being watched over, and looked after.

More words seemed to form themselves in my mind. I understood that Timmy had not fully entered his body at birth. He was now having an opportunity to enter it more fully. And I was having an opportunity to witness this.

The next morning I felt obscurely happy. The dream was certainly strange, but it had felt reassuring. I kept looking at Timmy, trying to spot any difference in him. He looked exactly the same, but he was calm and settled. One might say he seemed very much at ease in his body.

And of course I wondered about the figures of light. Were they what one might call angels? They weren't human, as such. I saw them as elongated figures made out of light. But somehow being with them made me feel good. Even writing about them now makes me feel good.

If there are healing angels, they had surely been with Tim while he slept.

Falling for the 'miracle cure'

There was no overnight change in Timmy. However, over the following weeks he started blooming and putting on weight, in the way that babies do. Pictures from a holiday we took in the Lake District show a baby who looks perfectly healthy, even though he still couldn't sit up on his own. He was eight months old at that time.

The chromosome test, like all the other tests, came back negative. We'd seen a geneticist who said she was sure his problems did not have a genetic cause. She said there were several syndromes he could have belonged to, but his apparent brightness meant he didn't fit in with any of them. It would be many years before genetic testing reached the point of giving us answers about Timmy's genetic code.

At a routine appointment with his paediatric consultant she said, "He's really come on. I've been watching him and socially he seems very 'together'."

At this stage, he was still being breastfed. He had taken well to puréed foods. He had never had a single illness beyond mild colds.

And then, disaster struck.

It came in the guise of more medical intervention. Some months previously, we had asked for Timmy to be referred to Great Ormond Street Hospital in London. We did this, ironically, because we felt the testing had got out of hand. We thought we stood a better chance of getting definitive answers at what we believed to be one of the world's best hospitals for children.

And we *were* still looking for answers. Timmy's head was noticeably smaller than it should be. This is known as microcephaly. It's not a diagnosis, just a description – the word comes from the Greek for 'small head'.

At Great Ormond Street, we first met a rather wonderful neurosurgeon who laid his tapering fingers over Timmy's unusually small skull and boomed, "This child is not a candidate for my work."

He then explained that this was not necessarily a good thing for Timmy. His skull was healthy. It just wasn't growing as fast as it should because his brain wasn't growing fast. *That* was the problem: why wasn't his brain growing?

We then met a neurologist whom Steven and I both

immediately liked. She was quite excited about Timmy. After asking a few questions she was almost certain that he had an extremely rare metabolic disorder. The gist of it was that he probably wasn't absorbing one of the B vitamins: biotin.

A blood test would prove it one way or another. In the meantime, she wanted him to start immediately on megadoses of biotin, because it couldn't do any harm, and she was sure it was the answer.

We'd never heard of biotin. Afterwards, I looked it up. It's one of the lesser-known B-vitamins, and it's essential for metabolizing carbohydrates, proteins and fats. It helps with general growth. The body requires tiny quantities. Bacteria in the gut manufacture it, so deficiency is highly unusual. However, antibiotics can wipe out the bacteria that produce it.

Symptoms include lack of hair and poor skin. Timmy didn't have much hair, but this isn't unusual in blond babies. His skin has always been very good. We considered these facts and then dismissed them, in the interests of a miracle cure. After all, we told ourselves, he did have antibiotics at birth, and he'd also had some for a few months as a prophylactic for the kidney anomaly he'd been born with.

We were also impressed by the Great Ormond Street label. Surely here we would find the answers we were seeking?

For three weeks, we fed Timmy biotin in enormous doses that you can't get through a GP's prescription. We had to obtain it directly from Great Ormond Street. For three weeks, Timmy had frequent diarrhoea. We were very concerned about that. I rang the neurologist who said, "It can't be the biotin. Do please continue with the course and we should see some positive results very quickly."

After three weeks the blood test eventually came back. It was negative. Timmy did not have biotin deficiency. We stopped the biotin, and the diarrhoea also stopped.

Two days later, Timmy developed a raging ear infection, so

bad that he had to go into hospital overnight. That infection ran into an upper respiratory infection, and another, and another.

From October till December during Timmy's first year, he was never fully well. By the end of December, he was extremely poorly. On the day before New Year's Eve, a fortnight before his second birthday, he was admitted to hospital with respiratory syncytial virus and secondary pneumonia. He was put into a side room, on his own – a tacit admission that his case was serious.

Timmy spent ten days in an oxygen tent. He was pumped intravenously with antibiotics. He stopped eating, drinking, even breastfeeding. He was put on a drip. The drip leaked into his arm and made it blow up like a balloon. This clearly hurt him, but he didn't have much strength to cry. After that episode he was fed via a nasogastric tube and he lay quietly, pale and yellow, inside his oxygen tent. He was nothing like his usual lively self.

During this time, there was another frightening development. Our baby had been born with a beautifully straight back. But in the illnesses leading up to the pneumonia, his spine began to develop a curvature. And in the fortnight he was in hospital it grew noticeably worse. We saw X-rays that clearly showed this.

We gazed down at our much-loved baby in his oxygen tent and felt fear. It seemed as though he was falling to pieces before our eyes. And there was nothing we could do about it, except pray.

5. Hospital

I don't often go back to Queen Mary's Hospital, where Tim was born, and where many of the tests took place. It's become a rather ghostly version of its old self. It's quieter, and emptier, with fewer people walking along the corridors. You can't have a baby there anymore. Many other wards, including the children's ward, have closed.

It's tempting to view this fading hospital as a symbol of a wider malaise in the medical system.

A few months ago, however, I did return. Timmy and I were there to see an occupational therapist.

A journey down the long corridors of Queen Mary's is like a walk through the early parts of Timmy's life.

We go in through the main entrance. I am pushing Tim in his buggy.

"Hello," I say to the newsagent who used to sell me newspapers and chocolate.

"Business is not good," he says, shaking his head over all the closed wards. "Your son, is he better now?"

"He's doing well," I say. Then I continue to push Timmy in his buggy along the corridor, past the door on the left leading to the maternity and labour wards, now empty and silent. Memories of feeling powerless and worried come seeping back, together with that sense of wonder still: the miracle of a new child.

"That's where you were born, down there," I say to Timmy. He looks interestedly in the right direction, but I have no idea how much he understands. At three, he still only has a few words, which come and go.

We continue past the chapel where I went in and prayed during the worst times. Steven spent quiet moments there too. It was always such a silent room. I never saw anyone else go in.

Then, on the left, we pass the nuclear medicine department.

Through that door it's dimly lit and frankly scary. That's where Timmy had radioactive dye injected up into his penis, into his urethra. It feels almost as though I can sense the ghosts of our previous selves there: helpless, terrified, and deeply upset.

Still pushing Timmy in his buggy, I come to a bend in the corridor. Here, I glance left into unlit, empty rooms. That's where I went for pre-pregnancy ultra-scans and blood tests. I also went there for Timmy's post-natal scan. They were kind people, not too scary. Timmy always looked like a perfect baby in the prenatal scans. However, we did know in the last few weeks that he was small for dates, as they say. We also learned then that his kidneys had some kind of anomaly.

I turn right, and push Timmy in his buggy along the empty corridors to the children's outpatient department. On my left, I can look across into the windows of the old children's ward. I recognise Timmy's old window. The memories flood back, of that fortnight when he lay there, pale and yellow, in his oxygen tent.

To my surprise, they are not entirely bad memories. Something good happened there. A team of kind nurses looked after him. This meant that Steven and I, amazingly, had time for us. During this first year we had got on as badly as any two people can. We had spent progressively less time together.

In a strange way, Timmy's hospital illness turned out to be good for our relationship. It gave us time to talk and even to go out together again.

In the evenings we often went out, to see a film or have a meal. We reasoned that we had an unbeatable team of babysitters taking care of Timmy. We spent New Year's Eve having dinner in a really sweet restaurant on the Sheen Road, and came back in time to drink a fizzy non-alcoholic drink beside our sleeping child's cot.

Steven and I grew closer during that fortnight. It was a wonderful opportunity to step outside our normal lives and catch our breaths. Although we were desperately worried about Timmy, it was also possible to feel pleasure in going out. And it was wonderful to spend quiet hours in Timmy's room and talk about where we were heading as a family.

Change of approach

During this period we came to an important decision. We decided that orthodox medical methods were valuable and to be appreciated in a crisis situation, such as Timmy's current acute illness. However, there was no proof that they worked on a long-term basis. Some medical interventions appeared to have actually done more harm than good. Every medical test had involved pain, discomfort and fear for our little boy. And they had turned out to be futile. We had learned nothing from them that would actually help our baby – not a single thing.

I was pretty sure that the megadoses of biotin from Great Ormond Street had caused the diarrhoea. That meant, in its turn, that Timmy wasn't absorbing food properly, which had lowered his immunity. Although Steven was less convinced, he was very open to a new approach. But what, exactly?

We mulled over this question for a few more days. Timmy continued to lie pale and listless in his cot. His illness seemed to be under control, but he wasn't getting better. He coughed up huge quantities of phlegm, and everyone said this was good, that he was clearing it from his lungs.

One day, the head of the ward, a nurse called Ruth, found me crying in his room.

"How can we help?" she asked.

Her question made me think. "It may sound selfish," I said. "But one of the things that's bugging me is that I'm not getting my writing done. I've got deadlines to meet and I don't see how I can do it."

It wasn't really about the deadlines. I could have made an excuse in the circumstances. The editors concerned would have understood. It was more that I just needed some space to call my own, to write in.

Ruth looked at me, considering. She knew what I was talking about. I had been staying night and day with Timmy in his room. One Thursday I had dared to go home for a few hours. But as soon as I arrived at home, I received a phone call from the ward.

"Timothy's been a naughty boy," said the nurse at the other end. "His heart rate has dropped. It's probably nothing to worry about, but we think it's best if you come in again."

So I had returned, full of fear. Steven had arrived as soon as he could. Timmy's heartbeat stayed low for a few hours, while he slept. And then, it returned to its normal range. That was the most worrying episode in this illness. It was the time we most had to face the idea of losing him.

"Let's think about this," said Ruth. "Would you be able to do your work if we could give you an office, with a desk and a phone?"

I stared. "How would that be possible?"

"Well, you could have an empty cubicle, and a table, and we could wheel a payphone in for your use while you're working."

I could have hugged Ruth. I was very grateful to her. She understood that it's important to care for the whole family, because that helps the child.

So Steven brought in a palmtop computer and my files. In my little cubicle office I made phone calls, and tapped in words, and felt obscurely comforted by this attempt to continue my work. Many times a day I'd walk across the corridor to Timmy's cubicle. I'd have papers tucked under my arm to read by his cot. Altogether, I was feeling more like myself.

My body language also changed subtly, which created confusion on at least one occasion. That morning as I was sitting typing in my cubicle office, I got word that the ward round had begun and the doctors had almost reached Timmy. I walked briskly back, squeezed past the medical group and stood next to my baby's cot.

"Where's Timothy's mother?" asked the consultant. She gazed around at the circle of young doctors around her.

"I'm here," I said, wondering why she hadn't spotted me.

She did a double take. "Good heavens, you're beginning to look like one of us," she exclaimed.

That taught me a valuable lesson: in hospital, do not dress and act as though you are a scared, demoralised parent. In a very relaxed way, dress like a professional. You will feel much better, and doctors will respond to you as an equal.

Shining souls

One of the hospital workers who stays in my mind was a cleaner. I wish I could remember her name. She was from Africa. She always asked after Timmy. She always said, "Praise the Lord!" whenever there was any good news.

I think she prayed for all the children in the ward, considered it part of her job, almost. She always told me Timmy would be fine. Did it help? Yes, it did. It felt comforting, like we were getting real support from her kindness.

During Timmy's illness we also encountered a teenaged girl with very complex health problems. Of course, I had met plenty of disabled children in hospital waiting rooms during the previous year. I'd met others through our local special needs centre. But Bella, as I shall call her, was different. Bella and her mother both taught me a lot – not by anything that they did, exactly, just by being themselves.

When we arrived, Bella was in the main ward. I had to walk past her every time I went between Timmy's room and my 'office'. At first, I found her quite disturbing. I felt ashamed of my reaction. Her body seemed twisted. Her legs were extremely thin, as only the legs of a person who has never stood can be.

I never heard Bella talk, but she did groan, frequently. I wanted to make eye contact as I walked past, but I never managed it. So I smiled at her anyway, and smiled at her mother when I saw her.

Twice, over a cup of tea in the corridor, Bella's mother and I talked.

"When she was born, the doctors told us she would never leave the hospital," she said. "Well, she proved them wrong then, and she's proved them wrong many times since."

What absolutely shone through was the mother's love for her daughter. Her devotion and courage made a deep impression on me. And I felt sure that it wasn't one way: she also, I believed, received bucket loads of love from her daughter.

Bella had pneumonia, like Timmy. Over the next few days she became a lot worse. She was moved into the little room next to Timmy's. At first, we could hear her muffled groans through the thin wall. But then, one day, they stopped.

The atmosphere changed. When we asked after her, the nurses said they weren't allowed to discuss other patients. We knew what that meant. Large numbers of people visited Bella every day. I was struck by how many people knew and loved her. I added my hopes and prayers to theirs. I was already praying that Timmy would get better. Now I also prayed that Bella would recover.

Meanwhile, we had our own worrying to do. We were trying to jolt Timmy into recovery. I put lavender and lemon oils on tissue paper on the radiator. The nurses commented on the beautiful fragrance in the room.

Then I borrowed a tape recorder from the playroom. I started playing music non-stop: a few children's rhymes, and lots of classical music.

And Timmy suddenly did recover. In the space of 24 hours he was playing in his bed, and his oxygen levels shot up.

He was going to be okay.

I wrote about that day in my diary.

It's 7.53am on Thursday, 9th January '97. This morning is a good morning, because Timmy has been awake and alert since 5am. Now he is sitting in his upright oxygen tent, playing with a few toys. I've put on Vivaldi's Flute Concertos, *and freshened the room with lemon essential oil.*

The monitor, beside me, has two glowing green screens. One, on the left, shows the signal picked up from the probe on his toe. It's a series of peaks and valleys, constantly changing according to the strength of the signal. So it looks like a series of mountain landscapes, some evenly spaced, some towering over flat bits, some lowland plains.

The screen on the right reads 94 and 138 at the moment. The first figure is the oxygen saturation level in his blood, and 94 is quite good, though 99–100 is what we're aiming for. It often dips to the 80s, though overall it's getting higher.

138 is his pulse rate, which is okay. It goes up and down quite a lot, but always in the normal range. Except last Thursday, when we had that scare.

He's on the mend. Basically, we're dealing with the aftermath of the infections. He's full of phlegm, which he coughs up. There's so much of it.

At the same time that I was writing this, against all the odds, the groans started up again next door. Later that day I bumped into Bella's mother in the corridor. She apologised for the noise her daughter was making.

"There's nothing to be sorry about," I assured her. "We were so pleased to hear her again. Her voice sounds so strong. She's going to be okay."

And she was. I am left with the memory of a child who couldn't walk or talk, who had complex problems, who nevertheless attracted a constant stream of visitors, and the purest, strongest love from her family. That love visibly sustained her, helping her to recover on that occasion.

It seemed to me that those who met Bella and came to know

her benefited in some intangible way.

The next day, we were out of that hospital, driving home across Richmond Park, smelling the sweetness of the air and knowing how good it is to be alive.

It was going to be a long, long time before Timmy really recovered from that winter's illness, but circumstances were at last shifting in his favour.

During Timmy's run-up to pneumonia I had twice taken him to see an osteopath. But once Timmy was finally out of hospital, I took him on a regular basis. That was the start of our new approach. It felt like a good decision, but only time would tell.

6. Soldiers and Indians

When Timmy started getting infections that first autumn, before he went into hospital, I took him to his GP. We saw a new, young doctor. He shuffled through Timmy's enormous file of notes and looked frankly out of his depth.

"With a case as complex as this, it's best to take him directly to hospital," he said.

At that point Timmy wasn't particularly ill. He basically had a heavy cold. I felt let down. "I just want you to listen to his chest," I protested. So the young GP did, and that time Timmy's chest was clear, but the episode worried me. I resolved to change doctors, to someone who would better look after his interests.

However, something useful did come out of that visit. In the waiting room I had seen a notice about osteopathy sessions you could book at the surgery. I asked the young doctor about it. He looked pleased that he could say something helpful.

"She has a healing touch," he said. "I think it would help your son. I would recommend it."

Up until that point we had not tried any complementary therapies for Timmy, because I was scared it might do him more harm than good. This was, after all, the 1990s, and complementary therapies were still very much on the fringe of acceptability.

In theory I was totally in favour of gentle alternative treatments. But when it came to a small, vulnerable baby… well, I just thought it was safer to put my trust in doctors.

But now I had a doctor's recommendation, so that was okay. I was aware of the irony. Even though I was disappointed by his lack of confidence in caring for Timmy, his words gave me the reassurance I needed. And so, I booked a session.

The first time Sultana Khan saw Timmy, she thought he was a typical forceps delivery: narrow head, rather pinched-looking at the front. She explained to me that osteopaths often treat babies for birth traumas. The soft bones of a baby's skull can get squeezed out of alignment at birth. Through tiny, almost imperceptible movements, an osteopath can help the bones to settle and align correctly once again. Fretful, crying babies especially can benefit from this.

It was soon obvious that Timmy's problems were more acute. He was ultrasensitive to her touch. I thought this was extraordinary, as it didn't seem to me as though much was going on. Sultana just seemed to lay her hands gently on him. Occasionally I could see her fingers moving slightly, but that was all.

When Sultana laid her hands on his head, he freaked out, arching his back and crying. Sultana was gentle, and didn't persist. Afterwards, he seemed calmer, but that was all.

We had another, similar session. But then Timmy got ill, and went into hospital. We didn't see her again until the New Year, just as Timmy was turning two. From this point on, I started taking him regularly to Sultana every three or four weeks. I liked the way he seemed calmer after the sessions.

It was hard for me to tell what she was doing. Once, though, she laid one hand over the centre of my chest, and her other hand at the corresponding point on my back, and said, "I can feel worry there, but that's not surprising."

That evening, to my surprise, I felt incredibly relaxed, as though I'd been to a tropical island for a holiday.

In one of the earliest sessions, Sultana said she'd like Timmy to be seen by Stuart Korth, the founder of the Osteopathic Centre for Children in London. Sultana worked there sometimes and I think regarded him as a mentor.

So Steven and I took Timmy along to the Osteopathic Centre in Cavendish Square on a day when Sultana was working there. We saw many couches all in one big room. Nearly every couch had a child lying on it, with an osteopath leaning over.

Sultana saw us and ushered us over to an empty couch. She

pointed out Stuart Korth. He was walking from one couch to another with a respectful stream of osteopaths behind him.

I found the set-up fascinating. It reminded me strongly of the NHS, and yet this was alternative therapy. Stuart Korth was clearly highly regarded by everyone there – much like a consultant in a hospital. However, it seemed to me that the respect at the Osteopathic Centre was greater.

Stuart Korth approached us, with his little meteor stream of students behind him. He examined Timmy and spoke with his students and with us. Again, I found the language fascinating. The Latin names of orthodox medicine were there, but they were blended with an entirely different vocabulary.

The gist of what he said was this: he had never met anyone like Timmy. Our son's energy through his nervous system was seriously blocked. And he thought they could help him.

Then four osteopaths, including Sultana and Stuart, laid their hands on Timmy along his body, and made infinitesimal movements. Timmy freaked out. He clearly hated what was happening. I felt for him, and wondered if there was a gentler way, even though nothing much at all seemed to be happening.

After that treatment we didn't notice anything particularly dramatic. However, over the following months Timmy continued to have sessions with Sultana. And over a period of several months, he was becoming more 'together'. So it seemed to us that it was worth carrying on with the osteopathy.

Sultana also explained that osteopathy could help to raise Timmy's immunity, and for a long time he was surprisingly free of infections. He had no need of any antibiotics for over a year, which was remarkable given his autumn and winter of illness.

Remedies from nature
At this stage I was also just beginning to try gentle herbal remedies. I had already discovered that a few drops of eucalyptus, tea tree or lavender oil placed on a tissue and tied to the corner

of Timmy's cot when he had a cold seemed to help him breathe more freely. Or I might mix a few drops of one of these with a little milk and pour it into his bath.

On the phone one day, my older sister mentioned the herbal remedy Echinacea, which she had tried on the advice of a friend. She thought it was excellent for stopping a cold in its tracks.

I was still nervous of complementary remedies. But my sister had a medical background, and so did the friend who recommended it to her. Again, I felt reassured by the endorsement of people with orthodox medical experience. So I tried it on myself, and on Timmy.

The first couple of times I tried it, I slept wonderfully – a real, deep, healing sleep. Both times, I woke up with no trace of a cold. It seemed to have a similar effect on Timmy.

The next time I took it, however, the effect was not so powerful, though it still seemed to minimise a cold. So I continued to use it when required as part of my growing kit of well-being strategies.

Meanwhile, I was still seeing new benefits from the osteopathy sessions.

Timmy developed sticky eye, and it cleared up without any medication after a session with Sultana. I thought that was amazing.

We also noticed that over time he became less overwhelmed by sensory overload, though he continued to have problems in that area.

But in terms of growth, everything seemed to have slowed right down. His appetite never really picked up after that winter of illness. His feeding skills did not progress either. He still needed to have all his food puréed.

All aspects of his development continued very, very slowly. He learned to sit, but only a little, and only sometimes. He didn't like bearing weight on his arms, so crawling was a non-starter. In fact, he didn't like changing positions, full stop. But he did enjoy standing, with support.

The days and weeks took on a more settled air. The early feelings of shock – of living a nightmare – had subsided. Instead, there was an ongoing sadness.

Reading my journal from that time, I can feel the remembered sadness of that second spring like a physical presence inside me. Most of the time I didn't write about sadness. I was trying to be positive. I wrote about Timmy's various little achievements.

But I *was* sad, and the happy moments I recorded were like islands of pleasure in a sea of sorrow. There were lots of those happy moments, but they did not constitute a country.

And yet… through all of this I was still having problems with the double vision I seemed to have regarding my son.

On the one hand, I saw him as a normal, albeit unusual, child. I felt he was fully accepted by family, friends and neighbours. Of course everyone knew he had worrying health problems and developmental delays. But for much of the time they simply saw his vibrant character, his brightness, and his great sense of humour.

On the other hand, according to the medical world, he was a disabled, abnormal child.

Where was the truth?

And then, one morning, something shifted in me. It was just an ordinary morning. I looked at Timmy as he lay asleep. But then, unexpectedly, I could see the same face we'd seen on his prenatal ultra-scan – before we'd known there were any problems.

I remembered how our small, unborn baby had floated into view on the TV monitor, his face filmed from below like a cherub in the heavens. Now, 18 months later, I was looking at him from exactly the same angle. And, unexpectedly, I was experiencing the same feelings of optimism and joy that I had felt then.

It felt as though I'd been given a gift. I could remember exactly how it felt to have a normal, healthy baby. I treasured the feeling. I allowed it to fill the whole of my body, like a golden glow.

When I felt that glow, nearly all the trauma from endless

medical appointments and consultants focusing on Timmy's aberrations simply vanished. Of course we would face many more appointments in the future. But they never bothered me in the same way. Something had changed forever.

Some months later I was to read *Timeless Healing: The Power and Biology of Belief* by Herbert Benson, MD. I loved how Benson described that an essential component of healing is the act of remembering what perfect health feels like. He called it "remembered wellness".

Maybe, with babies, it's up to the parents to do the remembering. You can't force it, but if you can reach that point, you have a strength that the most pessimistic medic can never shake.

This was a turning point for me. From that moment I was able to build up strength and optimism.

Around that time I wrote the following entry in my journal. It's a little slice of our life at that time:

Today Timmy did two things that showed real progress. At lunch he was eating bread and butter with great gusto, which isn't new. But he was handling it very well and better still, I think he was swallowing some, though lots still came out.

The second thing was quite moving to watch. He was standing up by a chest of drawers. I was holding him under the shoulders, but he was standing so well, I could feel he was balanced. I moved my hands down to his hips, and he stood beautifully. I had the definite impression that he would have stood alone for a second or two if I had removed my hands completely.

I took a urine sample of Timmy's to the doctor's. Then we did our favourite walk up and over the hill, down through the hay meadow. The grass was growing high and the crickets were in full song. We walked through the Terrace Gardens, along the river and through the shops.

In Dickins and Jones, an old lady came up to me and said, "He'll

know me next time he sees me, I think. He was watching me closely
as I walked around. It's lovely when they're knowing like that, isn't
it?"

That made me feel so good. I love it when other people see his
brightness.

There were always little compliments and tiny steps of
achievement to keep us optimistic. But over time they never
really seemed to lead very far.

Timmy's development was always a little puzzling: forwards
a little, backwards a little. And yet, he was constantly studying
everything. He noticed all sorts of things: shadows making
funny shapes on a sunlit carpet... a tiny interaction between two
people... a picture that was sticky-taped to a wall that suddenly
came unstuck at one corner.

And often, while I watched him, watching the world, I noticed
something else. His able-bodied friends didn't see these same
little things. It was as if they were too busy rushing around to
spot the details of life.

Let me give you an example of the difference. Recently I
bought Timmy a plastic *Lion King* trainer cup from The Disney
Store. It was full of glitter and little lions that moved around in
liquid, within the double-sided, see-through walls of the mug.

Timmy studied that mug for ages. He pushed it this way
and that. He played about with the lid. He looked at his fingers
through the transparent sides of the mug. And he finally put
the mug down. I timed the whole thing. He spent *45 minutes*
studying that one little mug.

Later that day, a friend of his visited with his mother. I gave
the little friend the mug. He pushed it this way and that. He
looked at the lions moving... and then drank from it and put it
down. I timed him too. He spent *under three minutes* studying
that mug.

The mug was clearly as new to him as it was to Timmy, and

his mother confirmed that when I asked. But the difference in attention span was typical of many things that Timmy studied. He just looked at things, and experimented with them, for far longer than his friends.

Steven and I were beginning to acknowledge that he had an unusual brain. We started to accept that he might be an original thinker, whatever that might mean. It was possible that the results of his thinking might never show themselves. But that didn't detract from the fact that he was clearly documenting the world in his own, thorough way.

And yet, his doctors and therapists were writing "poor attention span" in his notes. I found the way they misread our son absolutely frustrating. Unless they saw him clearly in the first place, how could they possibly come up with the right treatments and therapies to help him?

Increasingly I was wondering if he'd be better off without all the medical intervention. But I was reluctant to turn away from it entirely. I felt there must be some good in it, buried under a lot that wasn't good.

Timmy was consistently failing every development test put in front of him. The textbooks I read said that microcephaly was commonly associated with mental retardation.

So where did our optimism come from?

Yesterday I came across a word written in a very old notebook of mine:

'operationism' – a concept is defined by the operations used in measuring it.

Timmy's undoubted skills were not being measured in the tests. Therefore, the tests found him a failure.

Near that word, I'd written another note, about a linguistic oddity I'd come across. It concerned an American physician called SA Cartwright. He diagnosed a mental ailment peculiar to Negro slaves:

'drapetomania' – the insane desire to run away.

So this has got me thinking: could failure, like insanity, be in the eye of the beholder?

We've never denied that Timmy has neurological challenges. It's as if some of the wiring just wasn't there. Connections have not been made.

Take crawling. Timmy couldn't crawl. His muscle tone was simply too low. But when he was a few weeks old, he used to move his arms and legs and crawl upwards over us.

Presumably he was using the same automatic reflexes that enable a newborn baby to make stepping motions, or a newborn deer to start walking within minutes.

And yet, months later, when it came to making the same movements consciously, he couldn't.

Or take rolling over. He did roll over a few times before he was six months old, like a good baby is supposed to. But then he didn't do much of it for over a year.

Language was just the same. Before he was a year old, he was saying "ewo" for hello, and "agoo" for yoghurt. But those words disappeared, and to this day he has no word for either.

At 20 months, I made a list of the words he would say. Altogether, I counted 24. Some of these he would use in combinations, like "dada bye", "dada gone", "my dada", "my mama", "my poon" (spoon) and "I good boy". But over the following months many of these, including "Mama", disappeared for a while, and new ones were said only sporadically, before they too disappeared to be replaced by another new handful, and so on.

In other ways, thankfully, he was more consistent. He was warm and affectionate. He loved hugs and would put his arms up for a cuddle. His sense of humour continued to be very visible. He would laugh at quite subtle things.

One day, for example, the three of us were getting ready to go away for a weekend. I was rushing about a bit dizzily. Suddenly, I realised that at one end of the room, Timmy was laughing at me. At the other end of the room, Steven was laughing at me. They were both laughing in exactly the same way.

At nursery and with other friends, Timmy was sociable. He enjoyed the company of other children, and little interactions with them. He was playful. He couldn't walk up to the others, but he had a very clever technique: he would just sit and smile at a child. Maybe he would even drum his feet in excitement, and the child would look, and smile, and come up to him, and a game would start.

Maybe they'd just touch or hug. Maybe the other child would give him something to play with.

At nursery mealtimes he would occasionally take food out of a surprised child's hand, or out of their bowl, and would do it with such a happy smile that no one seemed to mind.

Once, I sat him down at the breakfast table at nursery. He leant forward and dragged a big, heavily-laden tray towards him... and yet those same hands and arms had less weight-bearing capability than a newborn kitten. He was a puzzle.

As you might expect, he was very good at playing on his own, because he was so interested in everything we gave him. He would turn toys around and run his fingers over the place where the batteries were stored. If you held him up to the musical mobile that was suspended above his cot, he would lunge at it. But he wasn't after the moving toys that dangled from it. His fingers went straight to the wind-up mechanism.

Altogether, it looked to us as though he was working quite a lot of things out. But we had to be careful what we gave him to study, as he mouthed everything too.

When left to our own devices, we tended to treat him as the intelligent person he seemed to be. But every time a medical person saw him, they came up with damning expressions such as "unresponsive", "some babbling" and "poor eye contact".

Sometimes they'd talk about him reaching "his own plateau of development".

After such an appointment, I'd look at my son through their eyes and think, "Perhaps they're right. Perhaps you're not so bright after all." But the feeling never rang true for me. After a few hours I'd revert back to our usual ways: showing him interesting items, talking to him about all sorts of things. I took pleasure in letting him explore the world like the young natural scientist he seemed to be.

The wisdom of dreams

During Timmy's first year, I was busy simply trying to learn how to cope. I didn't have enough energy to be aware of where my observations were leading me. I still believed, more or less, that doctors know best. But during the second year, something in me began to change.

And my dreams pointed out the way.

On the surface, I was trying to be positive – trying to make the best of things. But that was just a veneer. My dreams showed me what I *really* felt. During Tim's first and second year, I had a lot of truly helpful dreams.

I began to notice that every time we said "yes" to a test that upset Timmy, my dreams featured dark, narrow streets leading nowhere. There were doorways too small to get through. There were other doors that were closed. Sometimes I had a key that wouldn't fit the keyhole. The key wouldn't turn, or it would break. And everything was up close in these dreams. You couldn't see far ahead at all. It was a compressed, urgent, miserable sort of world.

Pervading these dreams was a sense of sadness and hopelessness.

At some point in Tim's second year it dawned on me that

what I felt in the daytime was being reflected back to me at night, while I slept. *My dreams, therefore, were showing me that the course I was following in the daytime was unhelpful.*

I can't stress enough to you that this was an utter revelation to me. It had simply never occurred to me that I had a *choice* in how I behaved. I was just so used to trying to conform. I had spent a lifetime trying to please authority figures, whether those were my parents, my teachers, or those confident medics.

I was always quick to sense how people felt. From the earliest age, I adapted my behaviour to encourage good feelings in those around me. I was a people pleaser. It was routine for me to ignore my own instincts in order to please.

It took days, weeks and even months for this revelation to sink in. But gradually, new questions began to bubble up inside me.

What would happen if I stopped going along with what other people said? What would happen if I started to make independent decisions?

It was then that I decided to experiment. I was going to try saying, "No."

Battle lines

The doctors wanted to do an MRI scan, to gain a picture of Timmy's brain. The process was explained to us in simple terms. Timmy would receive a general anaesthetic. He would be injected with a radioactive substance. Powerful electromagnetic rays would beam through his brain, recording the presence of the radioactive substance, creating a map in the process. This would show any irregularities in the formation of his brain.

We agreed to the MRI scan. Timmy was booked in for it. But as the date approached, my dreams were truly dreadful: dark and constricted. The journey forward always led to a dead end. I experienced a hopeless feeling of nowhere to go and no way out.

It became obvious to me that I was developing some serious

misgivings about the scan. As the date grew closer, I realised that I felt so bad about it, I could hardly bear for our son to go through it.

But why did I feel so bad about it? Surely it was a standard procedure? It was time to ask more questions.

I learned from adults who had been through an MRI scan that the side effects could include headaches. So it wasn't a gentle process.

I learned from parents of children with microcephaly that the results of an MRI scan are seldom conclusive, and that scans could produce quite different results as the child grew older. So it wasn't a reliable test.

Timmy would also need to have a general anaesthetic, and that was a significant concern, to Steven as well as me. We both remembered how Timmy had fought the anaesthetic when he had his endoscopy at five months of age. We remembered how the anaesthetist had given Timmy nearly double the normal dose. And we remembered how laboured his breathing sounded for several hours afterwards, even days afterwards.

I shared my doubts with the neurologist, and asked her an all-important question: "How will it help Timmy?"

She told me that the main advantage was not to Timmy, but to us, because it might give us some idea of whether future children might have similar problems to Timmy. Even then, though, any results would probably be inconclusive.

By now I was getting seriously disturbed at the idea of giving Timmy an invasive test that wouldn't actually produce any benefits for him.

Everything became crystallised in my mind when the community paediatrician actually visited our house and tried to persuade me.

"But what difference would it make to Timmy, in terms of treatment?" I asked her. "We know what his areas of weakness are, and we're trying to improve them through therapy. Will seeing inside his brain make any difference to the treatment he receives?"

"Well, no," said the paediatrician. "I suppose it's just that we doctors like to know."

She was a nice lady, who warmly cared for children. And I knew she had put herself out to visit us. But as she was leaving, Timmy, who was supposed to be unable to talk, said, "Goway."

I think he knew what was going on.

That night, I had a dream in which I was walking along a broad avenue that led to the most beautiful view over spectacular natural landscape. It was by far and away the best dream I'd had for a very long time.

When I woke, I realised that the dream had shown me, without any doubt, that saying "No" to the MRI scan had put us on the right track.

This was a turning point for the three of us.

From that point on, the happy dreams regularly showed up. I walked through beautiful rooms filled with rich colours. I travelled through wonderful landscapes with wide open, soaring, stunning views. They left me feeling that we were going somewhere very good, that we were doing the right things to get there.

Sometimes negative dreams returned. When they did, I would review my daytime actions and make adjustments. And sure enough, the dreams would improve once more.

Another "No" concerned antibiotics. From his earliest weeks, Timmy had been prescribed low-level antibiotics to lessen the likelihood of kidney infection.

There was no sign of kidney infection. It was just that standard tests had shown that he had a horseshoe kidney. This meant that both kidneys were fused together in a horseshoe shape. We were told that this is a fairly common variation that many of us could have without even knowing it.

But there was a suggestion that he might also have reflux, meaning that urea entering the bladder routinely went back up towards the kidney. This meant that if he caught a urinary tract infection, it could cause a lot of damage to his kidneys. The standard treatment was daily antibiotics, to be given for the first few years of his life.

But I was getting worried about the constant presence of antibiotics in his body. They gave him mild, chronic diarrhoea.

So, sneakily, after a few months I had stopped giving Timmy the antibiotics. I felt terrible about this. I had tried to raise the subject with his main consultant. But I had received the adamant message that the antibiotics must continue – no discussion.

I didn't stand up to her. But I didn't do what she said either.

We met quite a range of consultants, over time, in hospitals all over Central and South West London. Whenever it seemed appropriate to do so, I mentioned that he wasn't having the antibiotics. The consultants all repeated the same message: if he had been prescribed them, he must take them. Then, during Timmy's second year, we met a new specialist who said he could quite understand our reservations. As long as Timmy had regular urine tests and annual kidney scans, that would be fine.

All the while the antibiotic skirmish was going on, I had a recurring dream. I called it my Soldiers and Indians dream. It was set in a rather wonderful place that blended early, pioneering America with the Amazonian Rainforest.

The soldiers were mostly old-fashioned ones, dressed in red, marching about stupidly. They were regimented, living by an inflexible code. In my dreams, they were slightly laughable. Sometimes though, they were thuggish and bullying.

The Indians were indigenous people who lived a natural life. They were connected to their landscape in ways I could scarcely comprehend.

I liked the Indians a lot. I liked where they lived – their wild, lush jungle. They spoke to a wildness in me that I scarcely knew existed. But I was also a little nervous of the unfamiliar rainforest.

The soldiers seemed more familiar to me. I was of their kind. Although I found them laughable, I knew where I was with them.

The soldiers had another layer of meaning for me. I grew up on military bases. Take me into an RAF camp and I'll find its bare simplicity oddly homely and familiar. Those bare lawns, undecorated square buildings, the vast, windy airfields defined at the edges by grass-covered bunkers dotted with daisies... home sweet home.

Each camp we lived in was basically the same. Home to me was always people, not a place.

Home was a bubble that moved from camp to camp, every two years or so. That bubble might also sometimes travel to dangerous parts of the world.

I was born in Cyprus, during that country's civil war. It was a dangerous time. My father lost some colleagues there, including one who was shot on his way to the local shop. My dad used to sleep with a loaded gun under his pillow.

My family moved from Cyprus back to England just six weeks after I was born. We spent a few relatively quiet years in England. Then, when I was four, my dad was appointed as assistant air attaché to the British Embassy in Moscow. Families were expected to go too. So we travelled with him to Russia, or the Soviet Union as it was known in those days.

We lived in Moscow at the height of the Cold War: on the eighth floor of a gated block, with a security guard at the door. We were watched by overcoated KGB officials, and we understood that our flat was bugged. People we met in the street were often friendly to us, but sometimes they would hiss at my mother. "Capitalist," they would say, because she had three children – my older sister, my younger brother, and me – and the Russians at that time were just allowed two. Abortions were state-sanctioned and commonplace.

We had a strange, fun and busy life of parties and play dates –

always with families from allied countries. My best friends were American, Australian and Canadian. We went to the Anglo-American School with other Western children... and right next door, the Russian children went to an entirely different school. We didn't meet at all.

So I grew up believing that the outside world was culturally different from ours and it could, potentially, be dangerous. But we would always be safe, I thought, inside our bubble.

And now, during Timmy's second year, my dreams were turning that thinking upside down.

My dreams were telling me that what is homely and familiar can also, actually, be wrong – even harmful. Conversely, the world outside the bubble might not be so dangerous after all, when you got to know it. Like the lush jungle of my dreams with its vibrant, indigenous people, the world outside might actually have much to offer.

It didn't take me long to work out who the soldiers reminded me of, in my present life.

The doctors we were meeting were safe, familiar, to be respected. But their code was inflexible, and it just didn't mesh with the natural world, the way the Indians did.

I knew my dreams were telling me to reconsider my views. In one dream, a spiritual and caring couple we know well, called Paul and Moira Cookson, directed me away from the soldiers and into the rainforest. This seemed especially meaningful as Paul is a godfather to Timmy. In others, the Indians helped me to escape or outwit the soldiers.

In one very happy dream, we were able to hide behind light, see-through gauze. We giggled because the heavyweight thugs who came to find us couldn't see through the transparent cloth.

In other visions, I entered the rainforest and relaxed in the warm, wild lushness of it.

Despite the obvious dream messages, I didn't want to reject the soldiers' way of life entirely. All through this second year,

I was fighting to reconcile two very different approaches to Timmy's health: orthodox and complementary. I didn't want one to win above the other. I wanted them to work in harmony together.

But the doctors didn't seem interested.

We started changing doctors.

The GP first. I went to a new GP and said, "I need a strong doctor who will be my son's advocate when necessary in the face of all these consultants and their tests." He understood, and has done exactly that ever since.

The consultant next. We switched from Queen Mary's Hospital to Kingston Hospital. Timmy's main consultant there has been marvellous. He has never imposed his views on us, but worked with us.

Just after changing, we got a letter from Timmy's old consultant, saying she'd fixed up some more tests that she didn't feel Kingston could do so well as her department. She clearly didn't want to let Timmy go. I cancelled the tests and sent back a note thanking her for all her help.

Changing doctors was hard. I found it hard. I wasn't used to being assertive. I didn't want to offend anyone. I was conscious of reputations, of people doing their best even if I didn't agree with their outlook... it was difficult. But I did it, and in the end it didn't take long: a phone call, a few words, and then it was done.

Meanwhile, another battle was looming. This was a big one. It concerned Timmy's spinal curvature, or scoliosis. And this time we were going to make a decision that would absolutely divide our orthodox and complementary advisors.

The worst day

Timmy's scoliosis had developed towards the end of his first year, during his season of illness. He was referred to a back specialist in Great Ormond Street. The appointment came towards the end of his second year.

The day that Timmy and I visited the back specialist ranks as one of the worst days in my life. Usually, when I was anticipating a bad appointment, I'd ask Steven to come along too. There were so many appointments – sometimes up to five or more in a week – that he couldn't possibly attend them all. So he just came for key consultations, and any meetings I thought I'd find particularly difficult.

But on this occasion I hadn't been anticipating any particular problems, so I went on my own with Timmy. The appointment was for around 10am, I think. We had to turn up half an hour early, for an X-ray. That part was okay, although Timmy hated X-rays because his body was invariably placed in positions that hurt him. He cried during it, which made me feel bad. It distressed me to put him through yet more trauma.

But after the X-ray there was a long, long wait. We kept being told the consultant would be coming down from the ward shortly. People were getting very fed up in the waiting room.

One mother I talked to had an older boy, of about 11. He was sitting on a chair, but there was an empty wheelchair next to him. Timmy wanted to go up to the boy, so I held him in front of me, letting him stand with my hands under his shoulders. The boy said, "Oh, he can stand," and looked away.

"Only with support," I answered. I had seen the yearning in the older boy's eyes.

The boy's mother said they'd been coming for years, and this long waiting time was typical. She said she invariably used to go home and have a long cry, although in recent years she'd got more used to it.

Many children in the waiting room had stiff, thickened bodies. After a while I realised that they were wearing back braces – rigid bodices that encased the whole of the torso.

Then I saw a back brace, being held by a mother. It was white. It looked to be made of rigid fibreglass, and it had a circular hole in the front over the stomach area. Somebody told me this was to let the child breathe better. Another person said it was for a gastrostomy tube.

I had been reading about gastrostomy tubes in an online support group for parents of special needs children. Some children have feeding problems. They find it hard to suck, or swallow, or chew, or they just don't seem to have much appetite.

Medicine's answer to major feeding problems is to find a way of getting liquid food into the stomach without the child's participation, through a tube that connects directly with the digestive tract. During a general anaesthetic, a discreet 'button' is built into the stomach wall, and this is then used as an opening for synthetic liquid foods.

The liquid foods are believed to contain everything the body needs. I don't see how they can, though. I don't think they contain probiotics, or bioflavonoids, or other plant constituents we may not know much about, which may be beneficial to our health. I don't think they contain *any* fresh, vibrant food.

Sometimes the gastrostomy can't do the job on its own. Perhaps the child is regularly sick. In such cases, a 'stomach wrap' operation may be performed. This stops food leaving the stomach in the wrong direction.

Parents usually find having a gastrostomy tube fitted to their child extremely upsetting, as you can imagine. But if it's being talked about, they're probably at the point where they're terrified their child may starve to death, so they welcome it, though they wish they didn't have to. They share their stories within the support group online.

After the operation, many parents find their child puts on a lot of weight, and they may progress in their development. But the weight gain and the progression sometimes tails off, and some children are regularly sick.

So here we were, in the waiting room, looking at all these back braces, wondering when we would be seen. Every now and then a nurse would come along and apologise for the wait.

Not for the first time, I found myself thinking that the nurses carry the weight of the hospital system. The nurses are the ones that do the caring, that say something small to acknowledge the fact that you are a human being, and it's not fair to make you wait.

We were finally seen around two and a half hours after our appointment.

And can you guess how long we were seen for?

We were in the consultant's room for around five minutes. We actually had his attention for perhaps three minutes.

It all happened so quickly. I found it hard to work out what going on. It was hard to come up with the right questions, hard to feel any sense of control.

The consultant was sitting at a desk in a corner, writing up some notes. Above him was a light box, showing X-rays. I presume they were Timmy's X-rays, but the consultant did not show them to me, or Timmy, and he did not discuss them.

He asked me if I was related to Timmy's father. "We're not married," I said, confused.

"No, I mean genetically," he said, smiling briefly.

"No," I answered, thinking what an extraordinary question to ask. Was he supposing Timmy's problems were as a result of inbreeding?

He asked me to undress Timmy and a friendly registrar or nurse – I wasn't clear who she was – showed me towards the couch, where I was supposed to lie him down. I did. Timmy lay there, waving his legs about, quite happy.

The consultant came over and said, "He has scoliosis. He will need to be in a back brace."

"How long for?" I asked, feeling shocked at the consultant's abrupt way of delivering this news.

"Until he stops growing. And we like to see them in their brace for 23 hours a day. He must sleep in it, just take it off for washing."

He leant over Timmy and looked at him as he lay there kicking. A note of surprise entered his voice.

"He seems to be developing remarkably well," he said. And then he was back at his desk in the corner, writing up notes, and the registrar or nurse said I could get Timmy dressed now, and I should go to the orthotist to have him fitted for the brace, and she ushered us out of the door.

And that was that.

It was certainly time for lunch by now, so I opted to take Timmy to the hospital café for a break and come back for the fitting.

After lunch there was another very long wait. It turned out the orthotist was coming from somewhere else, and hadn't yet arrived.

When he did eventually arrive, I was ready with my questions. We went into a little room that smelt of damp plaster of Paris. Again, I had to undress Timmy and lie him on a couch. Timmy was getting fed up by this time, and didn't want to lie down.

The orthotist explained what he was going to do. This was probably the first time anyone had explained anything to me all day.

Then the orthotist dipped rolls of bandages in a bucket of liquid plaster, and laid them over Timmy's chest and stomach. As the plaster dried, the bandages hardened, becoming hot and tight over him. You could see Timmy was getting uncomfortable, but he was still busy watching, trying to take in what was going on.

Then, when the cast had hardened enough, it was removed and put to one side. Timmy had to turn over on to his front, and have the whole process repeated. There was plaster everywhere by now: little bits of dust and granules. His face was on some of it, even though I tried to lift him out of it. He was coughing and choking. On his back, the damp bandages were drying and hardening, feeling tight and heavy.

He looked frightened, like a child being buried alive. I tried to reassure him, but he started screaming. His eyes were staring, terrified. He was very upset, and so was I.

Afterwards, while the front and back halves of the little mould were put together by the orthotist, I wiped off the remaining plaster as best I could with baby wipes. While Timmy sobbed and I held him, the orthotist showed me a catalogue and explained the back brace didn't have to be plain white. There were lots of patterns and colours available.

Flicking through the catalogue felt unreal, like going clothes shopping in a torture chamber. There were all sorts of patterns. I quite liked a dusty blue design, with little teddy bears on it. I showed the book to Timmy and though he was beyond anything, I fancied his eyes were drawn to a jungle one with animals. The other design I remember was similar to soldiers' camouflage. Neither of us liked that one.

All through this I was firing questions at the orthotist, all the questions the consultant hadn't let me get out. The orthotist was a bit bemused, I think, but he answered everything. Timmy would have to be measured for a new brace every few months, as he grew. And yes, he could show me the X-rays.

I looked at them. You could clearly see the spine, straight at the base, then curving gently at the top, like a subtle question mark.

I stared at it. "Why?" the X-ray seemed to be asking. "Why?"

I could see that the vertebrae were squeezed together more tightly where they curved.

Afterwards, back home, Timmy and I were both shocked. It felt as though we had been mugged. I was aware of thinking, "Why weren't we given any other choices?" Then I remembered more of the consultant's words. He had told us that there were no other choices, that Timmy's back would definitely get worse without a brace, and that it would either stay the same or get a bit worse with the brace.

But something about the whole day felt wrong. It was hard to imagine Timmy thriving inside a heavy shell. I knew I needed to find out more.

I rang my older sister and told her about it. She suggested that Timmy and I re-enact the whole thing through, using a doll to play his part in the hospital.

So we did. I got Timmy's doll, Safari Sam, and a box of baby wipes. I took Sam's clothes off, lay him down, and then laid several baby wipes over him, pretending these were the plaster-soaked bandages.

Timmy watched all this very intently and then, as soon as I'd put the bandages on, he snatched them all off. After that he reached for the baby wipe box, got out another wipe, and gently, carefully, dabbed it all over Safari Sam.

I couldn't work out what he was doing. But then I remembered cleaning Timmy with the baby wipes after the orthotist had finished. Timmy had enacted that part of the episode all on his own. It was the part he spent most time on: the caring bit carried out by his mother. I felt touched by that, and reassured.

The thought also occurred to me that despite his learning disabilities my son, at one year and nine months old, could do a nifty bit of role-playing with dolls.

I picked him up and gave him a hug. "The question is," I said to Timmy. "How can any consultant, no matter how qualified, see you for five minutes and make a decision that will affect you physically and socially for the rest of your life?"

When I told Steven later, he was in total agreement. "He's not going in a brace," he said, and that was that.

I started doing some research to back up our feeling.

First, I looked on the Internet. I found a scoliosis support group. It was fascinating. The majority of the people writing had back braces. They had suffered pain, and their backs had got worse anyway, and some of them had surgery.

And yet all of these people said they were glad they had the back brace, and the surgery. They couldn't see that the brace had not perhaps helped. They simply feared that things might have been worse without it.

I read their letters and realised something that seemed significant: *they were all motivated by fear.*

Those were the majority voices. But there were others. Occasionally I came across an account by someone who had opted for osteopathy or its near cousin, chiropractic. Their letters were full of optimism. Most of them still had scoliosis, but they were free of pain, and their backs remained flexible. One mother even wrote about visiting a chiropractor, who had completely straightened her son's back.

Next, I searched for second opinions, both orthodox and alternative. The alternative first. Sultana, Timmy's osteopath, had been treating him for ten months. To me, she had never seemed particularly bothered by his back. When I asked, she said she was focusing on the whole body, of which the back was a part.

Sultana wasn't keen on the idea of a brace. She took us back to see Stuart Korth at the Osteopathic Centre for Children. Stuart was amazed at the difference in my son. He said Timmy was much better generally than he might have predicted a year ago. He said to Sultana that she should be proud of her work.

We talked about the back brace and Stuart Korth said: "Do not put this child in a brace." The osteopath's view was that a brace would do more harm than good.

And then Stuart gave Timmy some treatment through his hair. I think again he was addressing the central nervous system, and he said I would see the difference. There seemed to be a sense of channelled focus and concentration. Timmy himself seemed very calm and at ease after the treatment.

I was very pleased to have Stuart Korth's opinion, and went to the next appointment, with an orthopaedic consultant at

Kingston, feeling fortified by it. But the specialist's attitude was broadly the same as the specialist at Great Ormond Street. She said, "Is there any chance we could persuade you to put Timmy in a brace?"

I said if there was overwhelming evidence that his back was getting worse over time, I would be open-minded to a brace. At that point I didn't know that braces for Timmy's type of condition would fall out of favour.

So Timmy stayed out of a back brace, to the alarm of his physiotherapist and other medical people. But my parents were totally in agreement with us, and so were our friends.

Steven's parents, though always completely supportive and full of love for their unusual little grandson, were more nervous. This was completely understandable: what could we know, compared with an eminent Great Ormond Street doctor?

But Steven's father John had a dream, in which he saw Timmy as a young boy, running along a country road in Ireland, which is where the family came from. When John woke up, he felt that Timmy would be all right.

John had a special bond with Tim that seemed to grow with every visit. The two of them would sit closely together for hours on end, playing simple games that made them both laugh.

A few weeks after the Great Ormond Street appointment, I received a note from the brace-fitting department to say the brace was ready for its final fitting. I rang and said, "Sorry, we've changed our minds. Our son won't be having a brace after all." And I apologised for putting them to the trouble, but they didn't seem to mind.

Looking back, I found the experience of going against doctors on such an important matter both terrifying and upsetting. What if we were wrong? But I felt I had no choice. Everything in me said a back brace was the wrong solution. Even if it did keep his back straighter – and there was absolutely no evidence this would happen – it would constrict his body movements. It might have had a negative impact on future chest infections. It would have made him uncomfortable and miserable. The regular plaster cast fittings would have deeply upset him.

And there was one other thing – this really mattered to both of us.

Timmy didn't *want* a brace. The experience of wearing one was likely to be an unhappy one.

Happiness seemed an important consideration for us. If you can feel happy now, we reasoned, that surely provides your best opportunity to create a happy future?

This wasn't the medical view. But it was our view.

So Timmy chose freedom from constriction, and we respected that choice.

7. Trail of the tiger

During Timmy's second year, Sultana kept suggesting that he have homeopathy. She said homeopathy and osteopathy work well together, and we might see more improvements in him.

"Yes, I must look into that," I said, rather vaguely. In theory I could see it was a good idea, but I wasn't in any hurry. I was still adjusting to the idea of complementary therapies.

As we all know, changing your attitudes is an unsettling business. There's a period between your old way of thinking and the new outlook that feels very uncomfortable. Our friend Tessa came up with an image that describes this well.

She said people are like hermit crabs. We find a shell that's got plenty of room in it. We grow, until the shell starts feeling tight and cramped. One day, when we can't put it off any longer, we leave the safety of our shell, and go in search of a new one.

When we're in between shells, we feel very exposed and uncomfortable. When we find a nice roomy new shell and settle in, we probably still feel uncomfortable, just until we get used to the new place. And then, for a while, we feel right at home, until we start outgrowing that shell, and it's time to move again.

Well, I was in the process of changing, and it *was* uncomfortable.

Eventually, not hurrying, I rang our medical insurers and asked them for the names of some homeopaths on their list. They kept lists of alternative practitioners who were accredited and had been practising for at least ten years. This satisfied my instincts for someone safe.

The insurers came up with a name: Dr David Curtin, of the Hale Clinic in London. I liked the fact that he was a medical doctor as well as a homeopath. So I took Timmy to see him, and he said, "You're very lucky that he's bright."

He then proceeded to tell me things I'd never heard before.

He said that many children with developmental delays suffer

from miasms. These are traces of old illnesses, such as TB, that may have been handed down through the family. He said that miasms could linger for seven generations.

He also said that many children with delays have toxoplasmosis. This unicellular parasitic infection can cause a lot of damage to babies in the womb. I didn't take much notice of this. I had been tested for toxoplasmosis during pregnancy, and the test had been negative.

David Curtin said there was a way of diagnosing all these things. It was called electro-acupuncture. It was commonly practised in Germany, but it was very new to the UK.

Although he had learned the technique, he wasn't at that point confident enough to diagnose Timmy. So he referred us to Adrian Lindeman, who had brought the process to England and was busy training homeopaths here.

So Steven, Timmy and I drove to Southampton to see Adrian Lindeman. We found the whole experience very odd – "Hocus pocus," Steven called it.

As far as I could see, this is basically what happens. You hold an electrode in one hand. Another electrode is pressed on points along the other hand. A very mild electrical current passes through a vial containing a substance, such as toxoplasmosis, distilled to harmless homeopathic proportions.

If you're free of the toxin, whatever it might be, a high rate of resistance is recorded. If you've got the toxin in your system, a low rate of resistance is recorded.

Adrian pronounced that both Timmy and I had toxoplasmosis. (Steven wasn't tested. He stayed well away from the machinery, eying it suspiciously.)

"I can't have," I replied, shocked. "I was tested for it during pregnancy."

"Nine out of ten of the tests for toxoplasmosis are inaccurate," pronounced Adrian. He proceeded to tell us in graphic detail how the little parasite is picked up through cat litter, garden soil, uncooked meat, or unwashed fruit and vegetables.

He said that once it's in your body, it can never be eradicated by orthodox means. It's not dangerous for most people, but human embryos are very vulnerable. The parasite can travel freely through the embryo's brain during pregnancy, causing all sorts of unpredictable damage.

And he said that although orthodox medicine believes it can only be transmitted to the embryo if you catch it just before or during pregnancy, the reality is that the parasite lies dormant in cysts and periodically erupts again – just like that better known unicellular parasite, malaria. So you could pass it on to more than one baby.

He added that toxoplasmosis is very common in children with special needs, and orthodox medicine is simply not aware of this.

He did, however, have one piece of good news. It could be completely eradicated through homeopathy.

We found his explanations off-putting to say the least. But we were willing to try the homeopathic course of treatment he gave us. For five weeks, Timmy and I were to drink mineral water in which I'd put a vial of the homeopathic remedy.

The five weeks went slowly. I found it difficult to get Timmy to drink enough of the water. I didn't know at that point that quantity of liquid isn't so important in homeopathy. After the treatment, I didn't notice any difference in either Timmy or myself. I knew we were supposed to go back to be retested. Adrian Lindeman had said it can take more than one session, and that there was other treatment we could give Timmy later, to encourage the growth of new neural pathways in the brain.

But I just didn't get around to it. The truth was, I'd found his explanations a bit severe for my taste, and I was still adjusting to alternative methods. But by now I was keen to give homeopathy a proper chance.

I rang Dr David Curtin and asked him if anyone else a bit

closer to us practised the same technique.

"Actually, yes," he said. "Adrian's daughter, Natasha, is based in Bedford."

So in December 1997, just before Timmy's third birthday, I took him to see Natasha Lindeman at The Tree of Life Clinic in Bedford. Did our sessions with Natasha make a difference to Timmy? I believe they did.

On the first visit, Natasha tested us and said we both still had toxoplasmosis. She said we probably had it very badly in the first place. I liked her gentle, easy explanations, and she suggested that I put Timmy's remedy in formula milk, which made life much easier.

On the second visit, she tested us and we were clear. After that we went to see her every three months, and she gave Timmy a series of treatments to help clear some recurrent upper respiratory infections, and to help his neural development.

Over the first year that he had homeopathy, Timmy had a series of small developmental leaps – all the more striking as he'd had such a long period of nothing much happening. But now, month by month, he was becoming generally much more 'together'. His appetite improved, and he was just able to cope with things better.

There were all sorts of improvements. For example, he had been very nervous about changing position. I think this was because every time he moved, he felt dizzy and had to sort out a whole new load of sensory input. So basically he preferred not to move very much. Playgrounds were the worst places to take him. He would arch his back and cry if he thought he was going to be put on to a slide or into a swing. But during the homeopathy he started liking them. He became extremely fond of slides for a while. And he developed a long-term love of watching other children on swings and slides.

During this period his hospital therapists were saying, "Oh, he's really coming on." The synaesthesia I'd fancied he had seemed to diminish. His eye contact improved. And his muscle tone was improving. Our boy was getting stronger.

It all took time, and there were side effects. Homeopathy is meant to be totally safe, because the treatments don't actually contain anything, except the energy traces of substances that your body reacts to. It basically kick-starts the body's own defences and helps the body to heal itself.

But it seemed to me that homeopathy is like fighting shadows. Even though a shadow has no substance, you can expend a lot of energy fighting it. And I wonder if that's what happened to Timmy. After a solid year of little or no illness, he was suddenly getting infections and needing antibiotics again.

Natasha felt it was okay to use antibiotics if there was a bacterial infection – an unusual attitude for a complementary practitioner, I thought. She added, as did Sultana, that it would be a good idea to give Tim probiotics to counteract the effects of the antibiotics.

So, very tentatively, I started giving Timmy probiotics. They weren't so common then. The first time I bought a bottle, I opened it and examined with some wonder the small transparent capsules filled with white powder.

I knew that the powder contained a million or more bacteria. I knew the bacteria were beneficial varieties that occupy a healthy digestive tract – rather as plants, insects and animals occupy a healthy forest. But, like many of my generation, I had been brought up to think bacteria were dangerous, so it seemed odd to fill my son's gut deliberately with teeming masses of microscopic living organisms.

I opened that capsule and mixed the powder in with some breakfast cereal, and fed it to Timmy with some reservation. He actually had thrush in his mouth from antibiotics at that time. The thrush cleared up within 48 hours and his appetite, which had been suffering again, came back. So I became a convert.

Journey into the past

During this time I was going on something of a philosophical journey, in which my ideas were changing quite radically. I was adjusting to alternative methods, and I was doing a lot of thinking about how I came to be the mother of such an unusual child. I had gone through so many emotions by this time. You could pretty well make a list of them:

- Shock – "This can't be happening."
- Anger – "How dare they hurt our baby?"
- Guilt – "It must be all my fault."
- Blame – "Maybe it comes from his dad's side."
- Despair – "Nothing will ever get better."
- Hope – "I believe in our son. I believe we are looked after in ways I do not understand."
- Love – "I love our son, and that's all that matters."

One day, looking through an old box of bits and pieces, I came across a folded piece of paper. I opened it and saw, to my surprise, something I'd forgotten all about.

It was a drawing of a tiger, drawn for Steven and me in India, long before.

It was just a quick sketch on letterheaded paper that a friendly artist had dashed off for us in the course of a conversation. The tiger was mid-leap, his mouth open in a snarl. The artist had signed his name: S Jai Raj.

The letterheading gave the name of the shop: Hare Krishna Arts, on City Palace Road, Udaipur. Underneath it said: "We Make Paintings of All the Four Corners of the Earth (on order)."

I smiled at that. It looked like a clue, like something out of a Tintin adventure. And then I remembered the significance of that time, and I felt a shiver of recognition.

That day had been the third day of a strange fever – one of the strangest fevers I've ever had. I got better that day. Being given the tiger drawing by a friendly stranger had coincided with my recovery.

It was hard to say when I'd caught the bug that caused my fever. Perhaps I'd caught it at the start of our trip. At lunch one day, in an old indigo plantation house on the outskirts of Calcutta, I'd been eating some delicious fish which, I'd been told mid-munch, earned its living by scavenging along a murky river bed.

I remember pausing for a moment, and then eating more. I went along with what everyone else was doing – we all ate it. The fish was tasty, like steak. I didn't consciously feel concerned. But now, reading back over my India journal, I find myself thinking, "I wonder...."

Then again, maybe I'd caught my bug in the covered market in Calcutta. We'd entered it to buy flowers for our kind hostess. The market was divided into various sections: saris, vegetables, flowers, eggs... and meat.

"The meat section was in darkness," I wrote in my journal. "It stank of rotten meat. At some stalls meat was lying on slabs; at other stalls, *people* were lying on slabs. They were just resting... but the closeness between the two different types of meat was quite disturbing."

Then again, perhaps I had caught my bug on the train trip down to Satna, on our way to Bandhavgarh National Park in Madhya Pradesh. Perhaps, though less likely, I'd caught it in the jungle there. We had stayed at the White Tiger Forest Lodge. This simple place consisted of little rooms on stilts above the forest floor.

A jeep was sent out before us, to locate the local tigers. Then we had travelled into the jungle on the backs of elephants towards the position of the latest sighting. In the late 90s, we didn't understand that riding elephants might not be in their best interests; it felt like a real privilege to spend time with such an amazing creature, who seemed to be well cared-for.

I enjoyed the feeling of riding the elephant, sharing the large sitting platform with several other people. We bobbed slowly between the trees. The mahout in front of us had an indefinable air of dignity. His black hair shone in the sunlight. There was an exotic scent of sandalwood and other spices that seemed to accompany us through the jungle.

We quickly found the tigers. One crouched close to the feet of the elephant, and stared up at us with large, hypnotic, topaz eyes. I thought, as many had before me, how beautiful and how deadly.

Steven wasn't riding out with us that day. He was back at the lodge, with a nasty stomach bug. Every member of our travelling group – five of us in all – were ill at different times. Curiously, we each seemed to have a different malady.

Later that day, while Steven lay miserably ill in Hut No 8, I sat on the walkway outside and wrote in my journal. I remember children were on my mind that day. Although I didn't know it for sure, a baby girl had just been born in England. In time, she would become my godchild. As a little gift for her, I wrote the beginning of a story, about dinosaurs and how the world came to be the way it is.

Years later, I would travel with her to the Natural History Museum in London, and look at dinosaur skeletons, and perhaps find another clue to my own personal jigsaw puzzle entitled 'The meaning of life'.

But outside Hut No 8, I didn't know any of that. I was just writing about dinosaurs, while Steven lay recovering in the hut.

Why rivers run downhill

Once upon a time, a very long time ago, when the earth was still flat and the sky was young, a grumpy band of dinosaurs ruled the whole land.

They were the rulers because they were the only living creatures in the whole world. Humans had yet to be invented. And they were grumpy because their feet were always wet.

You see, in those days rivers didn't run up or down, or even around in circles. The rivers simply lay flatly and thinly all over the land like a gigantic, wet and boggy puddle.

The dinosaurs hated being wet. Unfortunately, their brains weren't developed enough to invent something useful, like Wellington boots, to keep their feet dry....

I remember something else from Bandhavgarh: a village woman, carrying a little girl on her hip. The little girl's face and limbs seemed to have been eaten away in places. I wondered if she had leprosy, and I felt very sorry for her. I looked at the mother, and was struck by the expression of dignity mixed with pride on her face.

Maybe I caught the bug when we flew up to Agra. We were meant to go all the way up to Delhi, but three of us – Steven, an old college friend called Jo, and myself – jumped off the plane at Agra, to the great inconvenience of the baggage handlers.

The next morning, in Agra, we got up before dawn. We took a taxi to the Taj Mahal. We watched the sky lighten very, very gradually, taking its time about it. We saw the early morning mist rise up from the dark Yamuna River beyond. The mist encircled the mausoleum like a shawl, before the sun rose and tinted the building in rose petal shades of pink. And then the sun rose higher, and the Taj Mahal became white. I remember the building sparkling as we approached it. I remember running my fingers over jewel-coloured crystals embedded in its surface.

Or perhaps, just perhaps, I caught the bug at Fatehpur Sikri.

Fatehpur Sikri is on the road between Agra and Jaipur. It is a beautiful city, carved in the pink stone of the desert. There is no water nearby – why would anyone have built there?

We learned that it was built on the advice of a hermit. The emperor of the time was desperate for a son. The hermit said the emperor would get the son he desired if he built there. There was some water in those days – enough to sustain a small urban population.

So the emperor built the city, and a son *was* born to him. But after 14 years, the water around the city began to dry up. Everyone had to leave. The city has been deserted ever since.

The hermit's body still lies there, however, in a marble tomb. The walls of his resting place are made of white marble, carved to resemble lace. If you can say this of a tomb, it's a pretty place: light and airy. People tie their threads to the marble lace. As you tie your thread, you can make a wish. Legend says that the spirit of the hermit will grant your wish.

If you ever go there, please be careful what you wish for. It may cost you dear.

I tied a blue thread to the marble lace, and made my wish. I kept my wish secret, and my companions kept theirs secret likewise. You don't tell wishes, do you, if you want them to come true?

But I will tell you now what I wished for: I wished for happiness for the three of us.

When I made my wish I felt absolutely fine. But by the time we reached Jaipur that evening, I was beginning to feel a bit strange. The next day, I was definitely not right. I felt dizzy and sick. I couldn't stop shivering even though the air was very warm. Most oddly, I suffered from vertigo, even when I was just standing on the ground.

Jaipur seemed to me to be a bright city, full of vivid silks and strong spices. My feverish senses felt bombarded. Everything was too bright, too loud... just too *much*. Even the breeze hurt. The worst sights, though, were in the back streets. We saw little children playing among piles of rubbish, above open drains... the smell was overpowering. I was sickened by the fact that young children were playing in such an unsuitable place.

The next day, we made our way to Udaipur. There, we stayed at the beautiful Shiv Niwas Hotel on the edge of a picturesque lake. The air seemed clearer here. There was a greater sense of space. The hemmed-in feeling I had experienced in Jaipur – as though the outer world was converging in on me, compressing me, and I was no longer fully in my body – was thankfully no more.

So on the third day of my illness we were exploring the City Palace Road in Udaipur. A friendly artist drew a tiger for us. I remember at the time that he handed us the piece of paper, I was beginning to feel much better. And by the next day, I was fine.

Now, six years later, looking at the tiger picture at home in Richmond, I shivered again. I'd always felt the illness in India was significant, because it had developed within hours of making my wish at the hermit's tomb.

And the hermit was known to grant wishes with a twist.

A glimmer of a thought occurred to me. The baby blue thread I had chosen, the wish for happiness... I had always half-doubted that I would have children. I wasn't sure why this was. It had something to do with the fact that I lived very much 'in my head'. For me, it was all about words and emotions, dreams and insights. I didn't feel like 'wife' or 'mother' material. I hated the idea of settling down into a domestic life.

It felt as though there was something essentially singular about me. Although I was in a relationship with Steven, it had an 'off and on' quality about it. Neither of us wanted to get married, although I did love him very much. And I did actually feel that he was 'the one'.

I enjoyed my singular life in many ways. But by the time of our Indian journey I had come to understand that, deep down, I wanted to have a child with Steven.

The day after finding the tiger drawing, I was in Bedford with Timmy, seeing his homeopath Natasha. I mentioned the Indian illness to her.

"You could have caught toxoplasmosis anywhere, including

your own back garden," said Natasha. "But if you found the picture and felt it was significant, it probably was significant."

She added that the dizziness wasn't particularly a characteristic of toxoplasmosis. Most people simply suffer from mild flu-like symptoms, and many don't even know they have it. But Natasha had previously found and treated a rubella miasm in me, and she said the combination of rubella and toxoplasmosis could have produced those effects.

There's no way to tell, of course. Maybe there's no link whatsoever. But it did get me thinking about the undefined happiness I had sought at the hermit's tomb, and the happiness mixed with equal measures of sadness and grief when my son was born.

I was also just beginning to get the idea that I would experience greater happiness one day. It felt to me as though my heart had started opening when my son was born – and it was continuing to open.

I remembered a long period through my teens and 20s when I had cultivated a hard veneer of cynicism. During that period I felt comparatively little empathy for others. My energy was spent on looking after my own needs in a world I believed could turn hostile at any moment.

In those days I saw other people as essentially separate from me. Energetically, I was a self-contained island.

Meeting Steven had created some cracks in the hard veneer around my heart. I remember driving from London to the North of England, to meet his family. It was Christmas time. I remember looking into countless windows of the houses we passed.

Many of these windows had the lights of Christmas inside them. I remember thinking that each lit-up home contained a family, or someone who was part of a family. And then it seemed to me that every family intersected with other families, like a Venn diagram... and there were lots of these Venn diagrams, countless numbers of them.

It then dawned on me for the first time that all families can be seen as one gigantic family. We are all related.

For me, growing up with a sense that my family lived in a bubble, and the rest of the world was outside that bubble, this was a new discovery.

That sense of being connected to others is, I think, at the heart of human happiness. We are social creatures. Maybe the experience of being connected to other humans is even the first step in becoming aware of the infinite life force that permeates all living beings.

At the time that I rediscovered the little tiger drawing, I had actually been thinking specifically about happiness. I had been realising that all we ever have is this moment now. But that's all we ever need, because it's everything.

"My life is not perfect," I was thinking. "But I can choose to live it fully, and that will be a perfect way to live it."

At that point, I didn't understand the life-transforming power of that statement.

8. A better way

We don't know how Timmy would have fared without complementary intervention – perhaps we never will. A sceptic might say, "He would have done just the same, or maybe even better." But occasionally I receive a glimpse of a more negative and painful world that might have been our son's path.

Here's a recent example. Timmy's lovely nursery, Monty's, moved from Richmond Hill to Sheen. The new location is a long walk from our house. So I thought I'd start cycling Timmy over there. He couldn't begin to cycle himself: he's only three, and he still has low muscle tone, with a tendency to flop over on to anything that will support him – although paradoxically he is also wiry and lively in his movements.

So first of all I bought a child seat for my bike, and then I shopped around for a helmet.

I assumed that finding a helmet would be a problem, because Timmy has an unusually small head. I'd heard of other parents in the same situation having difficulties. So I rang the Disabled Living Foundation and asked them if they knew of anything suitable. The DLF is a source of information on all disability equipment.

A kind lady at the other end said they'd send me a list of helmets and suppliers.

While I was waiting for the list to arrive, I went into Kingston, and as luck would have it, I found a helmet in Halfords that fitted Timmy snugly, as long as he wore a soft hat under it.

Back home, feeling distinctly nervous, I bundled Timmy into the child seat and cycled around the block, just to try the whole thing out. Timmy was laughing away. He thought it was hilarious.

It was a happy half hour.

Two days later, I received the DLF's list of helmets and

suppliers. The list shocked me – absolutely shocked me. The list was a rude reminder that as soon as I mention Timmy's disabilities, he is perceived as someone who requires remedial equipment.

None of the helmets were for cycling – even though that was what I had asked for. Without exception, they were for two categories of use: they were for children who fall down because they have fits, or for children who hurt themselves deliberately.

Third on the list was this item:

Self-Protection Helmet 5-6-10

Made to measure, protective helmet enclosing the head with a caged opening for the face, made of plastic with an Evazote lining. Front and back sections attach together with zip fastenings.

Optional T-shaped device available which attaches to the helmet and enables a head pointer stick to be attached.

Designed for children who have a tendency to self-inflicted injury. Appointments for fittings required.

Price guide: £450.

I stared at this description with a sense of horror. I could feel that horror deep in my gut. Remember, I was a mother who was enjoying taking her little boy for bike rides for the first time. He was enjoying it too. But it felt, oddly, as though somebody, somewhere, thought we were wrong to be enjoying ourselves. It felt like a reminder that if you have disabilities, you are not supposed to have normal life experiences.

When the shock subsided a little, I realised that the people who made and marketed such devices were coming up with the best solution they knew to a difficult problem.

I knew they meant well… but it didn't make the description any better. It is a given fact that any child who needs such a helmet cannot be comfortable in their skin. Something is not working for them on a sensory level. The helmet was trying to minimise the problem, but it certainly wasn't addressing the cause. If anything, it was adding extra layers of future problems.

I have a personal expression I use often when searching for the solution to a difficult issue:

Don't add to the problem. Remove the cause.

Although I didn't really understand Timmy's issues, I had done my best to address their causes through osteopathy and homeopathy, and I was just beginning to learn more about healing, also known as spiritual or energy healing. Timmy was certainly a lot happier in his skin than he had been as a baby.

This helmet, in contrast, felt like something that *added* to the problem. I couldn't help thinking it looked like a movie prop – perhaps one that had been designed for the film, *The Silence of the Lambs*. It was also very reminiscent of a torture device: a human cage that fits so tightly that if you wore it, you would never be able to breathe and grow normally.

Please imagine yourself, now, as a child who has been forcefully placed in one of these zipped, close-fitting helmets. Imagine you are left inside your tiny, customised and expensive cage, probably for many hours a day.

How would it feel physically, and emotionally? How would wearing it make you feel towards the people around you? And how would they react to you? Do you think you would thrive in such a tight-fitting prison? Or do you think, just possibly, that the abnormal constriction around your face and head would constrict you in many other areas in your life?

The face is such a personal thing. The eyes are often said to be a window to the soul. Much of our personality – our very identity – is revealed through the face. To cage someone's face seems especially harmful for all these reasons.

Please understand I am not criticising any parent who uses such a helmet for their child. There must be powerful reasons for doing so. There are also many designs that are less extreme and no doubt do a good job. It may even be the case, for example, that a young person with a particular set of sensory issues, perhaps along the autistic spectrum, feels safer when their head is hugged tightly all around by a helmet.

What I *am* saying is that a helmet with a caged opening is not an ideal answer. There has to be a better way.

The helmet also gave me that sense of double vision I experienced a lot in Timmy's first year. On the one hand, we were carving out an increasingly happy, mainstream life for ourselves. On the other hand, it felt as though we were being pushed back into the disabled pigeonhole. And it seemed like a really uncomfortable fit.

I realised this was another example of conventional intervention potentially doing more harm than good.

Medicine is great at clinical trials, which no doubt show that 100% of children placed inside self-protective helmets no longer damage themselves. But medicine is simply appalling at stepping inside the mind of a child – working out how that child thinks and perceives the world.

Again, please don't think I am criticising parents who have resorted to these helmets. I'm more interested in interrogating the medical establishment, to see if they could possibly build more empathy into their solutions.

The child in need of a caged helmet probably has sensory processing problems, or they wouldn't be trying to injure themselves. Often, sensory issues may well be the cause of such delays.

A sea of sensations

I read a book not so long ago called *The World of the Newborn* by Charles and Daphne Maurer. That book really helped me to step inside a baby's brain – that's your brain, and my brain, in our earliest days.

When we were first born, our brains could not compute the vast array of information that our senses picked up. All the sounds we heard; the undifferentiated world we saw, touched, breathed in and tasted; the sensory feedback we received when we moved a limb, or cried, or drank milk... it was all a confusing, dazzling, scented, tactile cacophony. And as we had no idea of time, this disorientating confusion all took place without cessation, in the eternal present.

I had the tiniest taste of this when I had my strange three-day illness in India, four years before Timmy was born. It was not a pleasant feeling.

Gradually, as babies, we began to make order of the chaos. Patterns emerged. We learned how to focus on what mattered, and filtered out unnecessary sensations.

But children with neurological issues are not fully able to make order out of the chaos. The receptors in their brains may work differently, and incoming sensations can get muddled beyond conventional recognition. Children with delays are often ultrasensitive to certain stimuli, while they scarcely register others.

Their senses may remain muddled in ways that are unique to every child. So when one child hears music, for example, they might also see coloured lights. When another is gently rocked, their body might feel as though they're being flung violently around and the motion might make them feel sick or dizzy. Yet another child might find their vision becomes fragmented when a loud noise is heard.

The exact situation is different for every child. But for each of them, the world remains confusing, uncomfortable and difficult to understand. They may well feel less safe than the average child. They might develop repetitive coping behaviours to create a sense of stability in a constantly shifting world.

A thing about elbows

During Timmy's second year, for example, he developed an interest in bending and straightening an arm. Often it was the left arm, other times it was the right one. He would stare at the arm endlessly while he bent and straightened it. It looked like an experiment he was conducting, but it went on, intermittently, for weeks and even months. We wondered if the repetitive moment was comforting in some way. I imagined that Timmy was building up a lexicon of movement in the neural pathways of his brain. By establishing exactly what his arm did visually when he willed it to move, he was beginning to chart cause and effect. That in itself wasn't surprising – any child might do the same... but not for months on end. In Timmy's case, it seemed that he was also building an anchor in a sea of confusing sensory impressions.

For a while after that, he developed an interest in other people's elbows. He seemed to enjoy their intermittent status: sometimes they were visible and pointed; other times they disappeared into the straight length of an arm.

This had its funny side. On one occasion, the three of us went to a mansion that was open to the public. By the mantelpiece there was an alabaster statue of a young man, life-size. Timmy looked at it and laughed, and laughed, in his characteristic silent way. He kept looking at it and laughing.

We couldn't understand what was so funny about the statue. Then Steven realised that the young man was standing, rather grandly, with his right hand on his right shoulder, chest out, chin up, elbow raised and pointing into the room.

From Timmy's perspective, this was hilarious... and suddenly it was from ours too. We imitated the statue, standing grandly with one elbow pointing outwards, and Timmy laughed every time. But he was also watchful. He was learning something.

So sensitive

I've lost my copy of *The World of the Newborn*. It had been much loved when I received it, and disintegrated further when I read it. I think it lost its cover. Maybe, it was finally thrown out, or maybe it went on to a new owner.

One thing I do remember from that book, however, was a description of a door closing. The noise is apparently much more complex than we believe. It's not just the 'creeeek, click' that we generally hear. There are many more sounds and echoes involved. As a newborn baby, all auditory input would be registered indiscriminately. But as our young nervous systems matured we learnt to screen out many of the extraneous sounds. We actually became unable to hear them. So for us, today, the sound of a door closing is simple, and not especially noisy – except when the wind or an angry person bangs it.

Our selective hearing makes us blissfully unaware of many of the world's sounds. It's the price we pay in order to be able to recognise individual objects, rather than existing in an undifferentiated sensory sea.

However, not everyone learns to screen out extraneous noise. For many autistic children with ultrasensitive hearing, a simple thing like a door closing could freak them out. It might be that, just like a newborn baby, they can hear every single echo of that movement. To a sensitive child it could sound like chalk squeaking and rasping across a board, amplified to thunderstorm levels.

And if, as the authors of *The World of the Newborn* outline, synaesthesia is the norm among new babies, the sound of a door closing might even be accompanied by strong odour, or pulsating light, or the feeling of being rocked in an ocean.

The sound of a vacuum cleaner being turned on could be a form of torture to particularly sensitive ears. I've read references to that on forums for parents of children with disabilities.

Or consider the vitally important sense of touch. If you are over-sensitised in this area, the softest fabric against your body could feel like a hair shirt. Even a hug from your well-meaning parents might upset you and make you want to hide away somewhere on your own. Or it might make you scream. Your parents would in their turn feel rebuffed. Much as they would want to, they would find it hard to give you the love you crave, in a form that you could receive.

It's hard for an adult without these issues to imagine how children feel when their sensory processing systems aren't working conventionally. But recently I came across an unexpected insight in the book *Simple Abundance: A Daybook of Comfort and Joy* by Sarah Ban Breathnach. This book offers 365 uplifting essays on the theme of simple, authentic living. It was written after the author sustained, and recovered from, a mild brain injury.

Sarah Ban Breathnach was eating in a restaurant one day, when a ceiling panel fell and struck her on the head. Her senses became jumbled up, leaving her partially disabled for nearly two years. This is how she describes the experience:

> *My eyesight was very blurry, I was extremely sensitive to light, and even seeing the different patterns of the quilt on our bed disturbed my sense of equilibrium so much that we had to turn it over to the plain muslin backing. I couldn't read or comprehend words on a page. But the most disorienting disability was that my sense of hearing was affected. I could not listen to music because it made me dizzy....*

Some of that description could easily apply to my son, especially in his earliest days. He was sensitive to light. He appeared to suffer from dizziness when moved. He often sought out visually less stimulating sights. However, he always loved music.

Imagine feeling as Sarah Ban Breathnach did. And now imagine having to put up with regular visits from therapists who seem to think that all you need to do is practise the movements and you'll get there.

Please don't think I'm against therapy – I'm truly not. Therapy can be extremely good when it's in tune with the child, gently stimulating them at just the right moment to progress to the next stage. Timmy has had some excellent therapists, who have adapted their various theories so that they work well in real life.

Occupational therapy, to take one example, is becoming more concerned with the importance of sensory processing. As awareness of these issues increases within the profession, it would be nice to imagine developmental leaps in many of the children they see. The biggest issue is often lack of funding, with not enough training for therapists – and therefore not enough therapists to go around. Most OTs, as they are called, are not trained in sensory processing, and there is no sign of this changing in the near future.

But Timmy and I have also seen therapists who seem to follow the textbook at the expense of the child. Physiotherapy in its worst form seems to be stuck in a 1980s 'no gain without pain' mindset. After having witnessed many physio sessions which made my son cry, I cannot believe children progress well when they are suffering.

I can relate to this on a personal level. During those early childhood years in Russia, my parents worried that I was clumsy. In an attempt to remedy this, they sent me off to ballet lessons with my graceful older sister.

Those first lessons in Moscow were lovely. The class was large, which offered a pleasant anonymity. Surrounded by many other children, I felt free to practise the moves without fear of scrutiny. I found the atmosphere rather magical. The teachers had performed in the prestigious Bolshoi Theatre, and there was a sense that real, authentic ballet was being taught, albeit on a really simple level. The movements were fun to do. I never felt self-conscious. I was simply one of the crowd.

But then we moved back to England. My sister and I went for private lessons in the home of a ballet teacher. We practised our moves in her living room. The sense of authentic ballet wasn't there. Looking back, I can see things that weren't visible to me at the time. As a child, I easily sensed this older woman's unhappiness, which was ocean-strong in her home. But I felt the negative emotion was all directed at me, and I think now there was more to it than that. No doubt the teacher had personal reasons for feeling depressed. She appeared isolated from other dancers and from her own culture.

She scrutinised my faults relentlessly, and magnified them by her attention. I became miserably self-conscious and of course I performed more and more badly. Under her gimlet gaze, I felt doomed to repeat the same faults again, and again, and again.

The lessons seemed painful and impossible. I remember many times trying not to cry. On one occasion I couldn't stop myself. The teacher and my sister just stared helplessly.

As you can imagine, I hated those lessons. They certainly did not help me to become more graceful – quite the opposite.

However, that teacher did give me something valuable: the awareness that when we try to force a child to do something before they are developmentally ready, we do more harm than good. It's better to create a kindly space within which a child can flourish, rather being overly directive.

Babies don't learn to walk by being told which limb to move.

We learn to dance when we find something, right at our core, that responds to music and rhythm. We learn to dance when we allow ourselves to be who we are.

Sooner or later, the child with sensory overload will find their own way of coping. Some learn to 'switch off' all the signals. Mentally, they go inwards, and learn to react to nothing much at all. Those are the ones who are called 'unresponsive' or 'passive'.

Other children discover that a repetitive movement can create a tiny, soothing pattern of order in a world of confusing sensations. For our young son, it was the movement of an arm, bending and straightening. Another child, more commonly, might swing their head to and fro, or flap their hands, or clap, or rock their body. Yet another child might create a harmful response, such as face slapping or head banging, because it helps to blank out other painful stimuli.

If your sensory patterns are overloaded enough, the movement you choose may well be one that damages you. So then, medical experts, who mean only good, decide that you must spend your waking hours in a helmet with a caged opening for the face. They are treating the symptoms, and the cause goes unnoticed.

No medic was suggesting that Timmy wear a helmet. But they did want us to encase his body in a brace, 23 hours a day.

When I told the back specialist at Kingston that he was receiving osteopathy, she gave a thin smile and said, "Well, it won't do any harm." It wasn't a vote of confidence.

One year later, I returned with Timmy to see her. In the intervening period he had had regular osteopathy and homeopathy, both of which were addressing his health in different ways.

During our session, the back specialist initially asked me a few questions about his health and development, and watched him as he lay on the floor, playing with a toy. After a while he decided to sit up and I registered her surprise that he was capable of doing such a thing.

"He's a lot more mobile than he was," she commented.

Then I sat him on my lap. She examined him by eye and hand. "Well, his scoliosis is about the same, or perhaps a little worse," she decided. Then she got the X-rays out and put them on the light box. We stared at them. She turned to me and said, with absolute astonishment in her voice, "It's got better."

"Has it?" I asked, blankly.

"Yes," she said. "Don't you see?"

And she showed me how the curve was less. It was still there, but it was noticeably reduced. And the vertebrae were noticeably less squashed together.

She turned to me again and said, with the surprise still obvious in her voice, "You were right. You made the right decision."

That moment was beautiful, and yet strangely precarious. Even then, I understood that the doctor's validation would not alter any medical views. We would continue to receive no encouragement for osteopathy treatment. Timmy in his little steps of progress was amazing, and yet so vulnerable.

9. Baptism

Today is 1st of March: St David's Day. But it's also a special day in our calendar, because this is the first anniversary of Timmy's christening. This evening, we lit the candle that the vicar gave us at the ceremony. It felt like a blessing spreading throughout our home, up the stairs to Timmy who is in bed, tired out after his friend Evan's party....

And the blessing seems to be all around Steven and me now, as we sit together on the sofa.

"I remember his smile as he was carried through the church," says Steven.

Timmy smiled all that day. It was as if he knew the moment was his.

At the service, we sat in the front pew. A girl we didn't know sat next to us. Her mother was in the choir. The girl and Timmy played and laughed together among the prayer mats on the floor.

Lunch was in a pretty, flower-filled room at the Richmond Gate Hotel. My father made a fine speech with his grandson in his arms. Timmy clapped and hugged at appropriate times. Everyone appreciated the way he became a natural performer.

It was an unexpected christening. Steven and I are not churchgoers, although I do consider myself spiritual. Steven has been an atheist, ironically, ever since he studied religion at university. He had a Roman Catholic upbringing and even had dreams of becoming a priest. But when he attended St Mary's College in Strawberry Hill, South West London, something unexpected happened. He became highly logical and analytical in his approach. As far as he was concerned, the mystery of the divine, seen through such a lens, just didn't stand a chance.

I think Steven was probably rejecting the dogma of his upbringing. I've seen him, while out hill-walking, stop still and look at a beautiful landscape with a different expression on his face. The beauty of nature and the miracle of life are things that touch him deeply. But he doesn't relate these to the 'God' he was taught about – an external 'he-figure' of authority to whom we are all allegedly answerable.

I think Steven and I are more in agreement about spirituality than we sometimes realise.

So, we never planned to have our son baptised. Yet when Timmy turned two, I understood that this was the right time for such an event. The guidance came in the humblest of ways, inside a shaft of sunlight. I was washing up in our tiny galley kitchen while the sunlight streamed through the window. And I had a sudden realisation.

"Timmy is due to be christened and I haven't arranged the ceremony yet!"

I also knew that my older sister must be a godmother to him.

I walked through to Steven in the living room and said, "It's time we got Timmy christened."

"Okay," said Steven. He looked unexpectedly pleased at the thought.

"Just like that?"

"If you want to, that's a good enough reason for me."

At the time of our conversation, it so happened that Steven's aunt Norma and her son Duncan were holidaying in Israel. Unknown to us, they visited the River Jordan, where Jesus was baptised. Steven's cousin knelt down at the water and collected some in a little bottle. "That's for Timmy's christening," Norma told her son, "because Timmy is special."

At that time no one in either family expected him to be christened – he was well past the usual age. And yet, they collected the water. How *does* something like that happen?

Our parish vicar, Julian Reindorp, visited us beforehand. We both thought he was wonderful. Julian asked us if we believed in God.

"I find it impossible to believe in God," replied Steven.

"I have absolutely no problem in believing in God," I said. "It's not something I have to prove or think about. I just shift my perspective, look at life differently, and God is there, connecting everything."

I was remembering the blissful spiritual vision I had witnessed a year before Timmy was born. Tuning into that experience is like a spiritual recalibration. Afterwards, life flows better.

But I couldn't find a way to say that. So I didn't.

How many more people have mystical experiences that they simply never mention?

"I've never been so good at going to church," I continued. "I find the language and some of the ideas rather old-fashioned and off-putting."

Julian accepted both our views. He talked about the contrast between logical and intuitive approaches to spiritual awareness (which Steven and I were doing a good job of exemplifying). He spoke compassionately about the struggle of raising a disabled child. Through all his words we had a sense of unconditional welcome. He said a prayer, blessed our family, and put us in the diary: 1st March: St David's Day.

When Steven's parents heard about the christening, they were delighted. They said, hopefully, "Perhaps Timmy will come on after the christening."

Forgetting all the great strides of progress he had already made, I found myself hoping the same thing. And it truly was a wonderful day, with many family members coming to give their support.

Family support. It's such a force for good. Steven's large extended family turned up in its entirety. My parents and siblings and Timmy's cousins made it. We'd arranged for a long refectory-style table to be set up in a horseshoe shape, making most use of the space. Even so, we were crammed into that room.

Afterwards we all walked down the hill to our little house in Albany Passage and squeezed in, goodness knows how. Some of the relatives spilled out into the tiny yard. I got out the antique porcelain that my grandma had recently handed on to me: Royal Albert cups, saucers and plates with garlands of dainty flowers against a white background, bordered with sky blue and gold. It's a quintessentially English tea set that has been used at numerous family events, including my own baptism, so it felt lovely to be using them at Timmy's event.

We ate delicious fruit cake made by my mother and drank endless tea. The room was very crowded and I remember catching my mother scooping up cups and plates from the floor, here and there, horrified to see them in such a dangerous place. She was intent on preserving the family porcelain.

We all hoped that the boost of family support would help Tim to thrive. Ironically, however, he developed a temperature the day after the event. And it was the start of a new period of patchy health.

Only now, one year later, can we see the strides he has made. We watch the candle flame of his baptism candle. We inhale the fragrance of warm beeswax. We feel the blessing spread through the house. And one of us says – I'm not sure whether it's Steven or me – "He's coming on now."

So what has happened in the intervening year?

Many things. More homeopathy. More osteopathy. Everest. New ways of looking. The first reaching out to help others. Our little family growing stronger.

And at the centre of all these changes I have a new regular practice firmly in place, which we might call 'the act of listening to your own inner guidance'.

This is how it happened.

During Timmy's first year, I looked to doctors for answers.

During Timmy's second year, I looked to complementary practitioners.

During Timmy's third year, I looked within.

The doctors and the complementary therapists do still matter to us. If anything, they are now valued more. Because I no longer expect them to have all the answers, I can appreciate the answers they do have.

What do I mean by 'looking within'?

Intuition, gut feeling, instinct, it goes by many names... it's an extraordinarily powerful force, a compass in everyone's life. I've learned that it tells me, through dreams, when I'm on track. It warns me when I'm off track, or even, perhaps, facing danger. When I've listened, it has helped me to step my way lightly through trouble.

It's that niggling feeling, that little voice inside you that says, "I don't want to be doing this," or, "I'm happy." It can come as shafts of light, a sudden insight. It has been called, many times, the voice of God within.

If we listen to instinct, if we make a point of noticing how we feel, if we watch for opportunities that develop out of the blue, we may well find that a happier life unfolds.

There are plenty of mysterious aspects to it, also. What made Steven's aunt and cousin collect water from the River Jordan at the same time that I received the insight that Timmy was going to be christened?

At times like that, it seems that we humans are not so separate after all.

Learning to trust my intuition was not, by any means, an overnight thing. It was a process – one that is still continuing, and most likely will as long as I live. It's not a smooth process. I notice I often have a period of discomfort before a shaft of sunlight. Maybe the discomfort is resistance to the process. Or maybe, as the following story illustrates, the discomfort prompts me to ask a question, which is then answered by my inner guidance.

Helping me, helping you

One day, a few months after Timmy's christening, I was walking through corridors of dinosaurs with Timmy, and other members of our family.

We were in the Natural History Museum in London. For some reason, although I was enjoying myself, I was also slightly grumpy. I was looking at all those dinosaur skeletons, thinking, "Why did you become extinct? Why couldn't you get yourselves sorted out? What was your fatal flaw?"

I was grumpy because there was a clue there somewhere about our own lives, and I just couldn't spot it and couldn't be bothered to. I only wanted a good time.

And then, a rope barrier was lifted. A group of people – perhaps 10 or 11 of them – passed through into our area. They moved slowly. Most of them had white sticks except a few, respectfully shepherding them, who wore the museum uniform.

For some reason, as I watched their slow progress, my mood lifted. I became calm. The answer was there. Even if I couldn't spot it, I knew the answer was there.

I don't quite know how to put this, but there was a difference in the air around the people with their white canes. A spirit of love and caring surrounded their slow progress. The caring was manifested by the museum staff. Gently, they helped them through barriers. They led them to the skeletons of dinosaurs. They helped them to touch the bony outlines.

And the caring stretched out more widely, like a blanket of most uplifting, subtle light beams. I wasn't the only person watching. All around that vast room, people were watching, and their energy, like mine, became softened in the process.

And then, I realised: the answer lay in the caring. Caring for others is life-saving for all of us, because we are all connected.

It felt to me as though the people who need caring – those with disabilities – come into being from the vast fabric of all life because there is a collective human *need* for their vulnerability. Being vulnerable is at least part of their purpose.

Those who do the caring receive something so valuable in

return. Hearts that have closed through trauma are able to reopen.

And of course we can play both roles within a lifetime. I can be a carer, and at the same time be someone who is cared for. Even a full-time carer – perhaps *especially* a full-time carer – needs help from her wider circle.

This is something that is built into our DNA: we are here to care, and to be cared for. Both functions are sacred.

Later, when we were in the museum shop, Timmy spoke. As always, this was a rare event. His cousins were selecting books. Timmy said, "I want one." So I bought him a pop-up dinosaur book. He thought it was wonderful and, for a while, slightly scary.

After that visit to the Natural History Museum, I realised my view of people with disabilities had changed. Instead of seeing them as lacking something – dis-abled – I began to view them as having *extra* ability – they were differently abled.

It was as though I had been wearing a pair of distorting lenses, which had now fallen from my eyes.

Once, for example, I might have viewed someone with the outward signs of disability totally in the context of their label, or diagnosis. But now I was seeing a person with his or her own particular qualities. On occasion it felt to me as though I could see a very subtle, uplifting glow around them. At those times, it seemed to me that they had not forgotten something that other people routinely forget: that we are all loved by an unseen intelligence – that we are the sons and daughters of the universe, that we are loved by life itself.

And then, I began to notice that some parents of children with disabilities spoke about them in surprisingly positive ways. They talked about how much their children taught them. The parents mentioned qualities such as compassion, love, laughter and forgiveness. They talked about enjoying life, about living in the moment.

These parents made it clear that their lives were enriched by their children.

A huge shift was taking place in me. It's hard to overestimate the effect of this shift.

I felt like one of the first sailors, nearing the edge of the known world. Nearly all my life I had been aware of the hazy horizon. I believed that I could see, or sense, the sharp, frightening place where the sea, our ship and I would be swept over into a terrifying abyss.

The known world was the 'normal' world: the one in which babies reach their developmental milestones at a statistically average age; the one in which humans all look more or less the same, give or take a few minor variations.

The unknown world, the terrifying abyss, was where you went if you were developmentally 'abnormal'. I had been clutching our son and scrambling on the edge of that abyss ever since our son was born. Now, at last, I was learning to let go.

And when I finally let go... whoosh. Acceptance came in. A sense of freedom arrived. I understood, finally, that it was okay not to conform. I realised that the world would not end if our son never got a single school qualification. I also had a sense, increasingly, that we were somehow looked after. Spiritually, we were not alone on our challenging journey.

I'd love to say this feeling stayed with me. Unfortunately, it did not. It came and went. It was there in our own safe haven, our home. It was there when we went out and about in Richmond. It was there when we met up with friends and family. And yet it invariably vanished when I met someone from the public sector whose job it was to look after children with disabilities: doctors, therapists, health visitors. On uncharitable days I wondered if such jobs created the need to make a person feel 'less than'. After all, if Timmy and all the 'Timmys' in the world were without 'special needs', the professionals would be out of a job.

A lot of the pressure was subtle. I'm sure that all professionals we met meant well. So why was I left feeling diminished after so many of the appointments?

Let me give you an example, that happened just yesterday.

Timmy's health visitor came to see us. She came with forms for free nappies. As Timmy is now three with no sign of becoming continent, he is eligible for free nappies. I feel grateful for this service. It's clearly a help not to have to pay for nappies endlessly.

I like the health visitor. We get on well. She's been helpful and honest in the past. Once, I was resisting some test or other and she said, "I wouldn't have it done to my children."

But despite the fact that I like her, something about the visit was bugging me. It wasn't her fault: she was just asking the questions she was trained to ask. But her questions left me feeling as though I was somehow not quite coping.

"How do you manage about holidays?" she asked. "Do you take all of Timothy's equipment?"

"What equipment?" I replied, puzzled. "We don't take a thing, apart from his stroller. We don't have a problem with holidays. We go anywhere we feel like going."

My friends know that we are reasonably adventurous with our holidays: we took him on a boat trip along the Thames one week. Another time, we actually travelled to the Caribbean – to the island of St Lucia (more of which in a later chapter). Generally I like to think that I come across as an *able* person. So why was I beginning to feel like a frail old lady, being visited by someone more able than me? I didn't like the sensation. It was as if the 'real me' was invisible and unacknowledged.

The health visitor filled out the nappy forms. I signed in two places on Timmy's behalf. After she left, I looked at our copies of the forms more carefully. This is what I had signed:

I, Suzanne Askham, declare that I am suffering from a chronic disability, and that I am receiving the following goods which are being supplied to me for my personal use: Incontinence protection products.

I invite you to insert your name into that sentence in place of mine.

How does it make you feel?

Just to be clear, I am not suffering from a chronic disability and I do not require incontinence protection products. However, the form required me to say that I was incontinent.

No one, incontinent or otherwise, should be required to sign a form like that. It's demeaning and depressing. It's not conducive to health or healing.

For me, it felt as though I was being pushed into a disadvantaged box that I simply didn't belong in. Having to sign a statement saying that I was chronically disabled felt like a negative affirmation that could even become a self-fulfilling prophecy.

I could actually picture the official who designed that form thinking, "Let's make them feel bad, because they should feel bad... because they're DISABLED!"

I recognised my reaction of anger and injustice. That in itself was helpful. The first step away from the disadvantaged box is to 'own' your own feelings.

The idea of positive affirmations is reasonably mainstream nowadays. It makes sense that regularly repeated positive statements can help us to feel uplifted and can help us to move into a more positive future.

And yet the health service – which ought to be focusing on helping people to feel healthier – specialises in negative affirmations. If you don't believe me, go and sit in your GP's waiting room and read all the posters about smoking, bacteria and disease. It's not easy to feel healthy with such negative messages around you.

People often complain about the health service. We all know it's overstretched and underfunded. But this has nothing to do with money. It's all about attitude.

Is it about projection?

I touched on this subject earlier in relation to doctors who feel under great pressure to be perfect. I questioned where the parts of their psyche that felt like a failure ended up.

But the problem extends far beyond doctors.

In olden times, princes could not be punished because they were senior in rank to the people looking after them. So a prince would have a whipping boy, or scapegoat, who was junior in rank. Every time the prince misbehaved, the whipping boy would be punished. Although the system was blatantly unfair, everyone was satisfied that discipline was seen to be done. And some seriously spoilt princes grew up to be kings.

Scapegoating is a form of projection, in which weaknesses that belong to one individual are projected on to another – who then has to pay the consequences.

Psychologists today talk about projecting. We all have qualities that we choose not to own. We project these elements on to other people. "She's loud-mouthed, he's bossy, they're evil...."

I wonder if there's some kind of projection going on with disabled people in our society: "If they're disabled, then I'm okay."

And it's important to be okay, because we haven't been brought up to understand and cope with our weaknesses. Instead, we hide them. We pretend they're not there.

We haven't learnt the fundamental truth:

In our weakness lies our strength.

A humble place

The dream that I had on the eve of starting this book was about Timmy lying like a newborn baby in a manger. But he wasn't really like Jesus, because his skin was blue, the colour of someone who is deprived of oxygen.

I wonder if the dream was actually about humility and meekness.

Jesus was born in the most humble place imaginable: a stable.

He said that the meek shall inherit the earth. These words are beginning to make sense to me.

In our weakness lies our strength.

Children with health problems and their parents are also in the humblest place imaginable. We learn humility because others sometimes reject us or look down on us. If we're lucky, they feel compassion for us. If we're really lucky, they treat us as equals – but it's not a given.

However, if you do find yourself in that humble place, once you've picked yourself up, dusted yourself off and looked around, you may find there are advantages.

For a start, it's a friendly community. There are many people like you, whom you've never noticed before. Some are parents of disabled children. Others have struggled from an alphabet of other challenges: abuse, bereavement, cancer, depression... there are so many ways for humanity to suffer.

You discover there's something likeable about these other people who have found themselves in the Vale of Humility. They're not trying to hide anything. They're honest about their weaknesses. This means conversation between you can be unusually clear and open. Empathy flourishes.

You and many of the other people who live in the Vale of Humility have gone through a heart-opening process. You can all feel each other's emotions.

And then you realise why so many people shut themselves off emotionally from those in trouble. Caring hurts.

Every human being has been hurt more than once, during babyhood or childhood. I believe abandonment issues are a problem for every member of our society. I'm pretty certain that leaving a baby to cry, for example, is a form of abandonment. It's also a form of torture. The baby doesn't understand the concept of time. The baby only knows that it is in an eternal abyss of abandonment and pain.

However, we live in a culture of 'just getting on with it'. So we wall up the hurt, whatever it might be. Over time, we can wall up a very large number of hurts. A giant part of our psyche can become frozen behind these internal walls. Our hearts close up. Our ability to empathise with others shrinks. Our ability to feel compassion vanishes.

This is the norm in our society. We have people in caring professions who are wounded on the inside and they don't know it. Often they go into a healing profession in a vain attempt to mend their own unacknowledged pain.

It's often only when we go through one or more 'wake-up' calls that our hearts may open again. Even though caring hurts, we know it's worth the pain because it means we're brave enough to live life to the full.

There's another extremely curious thing about the Vale of Humility: the visibility is extremely good here. The stable that I saw in my dream is in a wide, open and fertile valley. There are slopes leading to mountains around, and ways through to other plains and valleys. You can see it all as clearly as a pilot flying on the clearest of days.

Why is it so clear?

Because we who live in the Vale of Humility have allowed ourselves to see. We are no longer peering sightlessly through a filter composed of all the things we suppressed before. We can see 'what is'. We stop being scared.

All right, we still get scared. But we spend much less time feeling scared, or negative, or hopeless.

Perhaps, for example, I look across the valley and see a solitary magpie, going about his daily business of being a harbinger of sorrow according to the traditional English folk rhyme.

"One for sorrow, two for joy...."

Once upon a time, superstitiously, I would have looked for another magpie, to attract joy rather than sorrow into my life.

Today, I no longer mind that just one magpie is present. Instead, I admire its glossy black, white and blue coat. I may even remind myself that sorrow can turn out to be a beautifully-wrapped gift, bringing me something I didn't have before.

We who live in the Vale of Humility are willing to see obstacles in our path for what they are, rather than pretending they're not there. At night, we can see the stars clearly, and navigate by them. The vast, sheltering night sky is our friend, and we sleep safe beneath it.

When you start living happily in the Vale of Humility, you start noticing something else as well. In all sorts of mysterious and unexpected ways, you keep getting help when you need it. The first time it happens you call it good luck or coincidence. If it keeps happening you might feel spooked for a while. And then, over time, you relax and get used to it.

Gradually, you realise that your new clarity of vision may not be so clear after all. There are forces that you cannot see. These forces have something to do with your developing intuition – your inner guidance.

Your intuition is a most amazing friend. It's your route to infinite help and wisdom.

Evolution of intuition

I was connecting with my intuition, and struggling with it at the same time. The logical side of my brain craved concrete, proven facts.

On a personal level, I was having some 'way out' experiences: radiantly clear dreams, the powerful spiritual vision that preceded my son's conception, experiences of subtle, glowing energy and sparks of light around people, my name being said by an invisible presence....

And yet I put all these experiences into a private box. They existed in my inner world, but not in the outer world of hard facts and analysis. And I felt the tension that comes from holding two opposing viewpoints simultaneously.

When Timmy was two, *The Celestine Vision* by James Redfield was published. I read this book avidly, and found it helpful. Redfield describes how religion was once dominant on our planet, until science took over. He suggests, encouragingly, that science today is being tempered by greater spiritual and intuitive awareness.

The world is a lot more mysterious than we generally let ourselves imagine. Science can give us amazing insights. But science is also constantly proving itself wrong. What was held to be a truth in the past may be laughed at today. What we have proven scientifically today may be laughed at tomorrow.

There are two tools that I have learned to use that help me access my internal world of intuitive wisdom.

The first is the trick of opposites. In a nutshell, this involves reversing the way you normally look at life. This is a quick, practical strategy.

The second is to access the unconscious realms of our mind that are normally hidden to us. This is a huge area, a lifetime's work.

Let's look at each in more detail.

The trick of opposites

We all have strengths and weaknesses. The trick of opposites tells us that weaknesses can and frequently do turn out to be strengths, and vice versa.

One historic example of this is the early childhood of Albert Einstein. He didn't talk until he was four. He must have worried his parents during all those silent years. Today he would be classed as a child with special needs. He might well receive speech therapy. However, was young Albert's late talking really such a problem? During his years of silence he developed his extraordinary abstract thinking skills. And all his life he enjoyed a rich interior world in which dreams were a valued teacher. So the perceived weakness of being a late talker turned out to be, in fact, a strength.

I love thinking of all the many children with special needs that I've met in this respect – including, of course, our own son. What hidden strengths do they have? What insights about the world, and human nature, do they enjoy?

One characteristic that Timmy has is an unlimited capacity for unconditional love. It makes him an absolute joy to be with. When I simply sit with him, I feel a wave of warm loving energy envelop me. I enter a state of great calmness. I become very relaxed. I feel as though I am bathing in a sea of acceptance.

Linked with this, Timmy also has an unlimited capacity for happiness. Although he has suffered more than many, he is so often to be seen with a smile on his face.

He also seems to have an uncanny ability to hear unspoken thoughts, and also, curiously, to know something just before it happens.

I was travelling downwards in a lift with Timmy once, in a department store. Suddenly, he let out a frightened cry. A moment later, the lift stopped between floors. For a few, unnerving minutes, we were stuck. What had Timmy perceived, that I had missed?

Learning to love the unconscious

The unconscious is the fathomless well that our egos fear, because we can never control or understand it.

But there is nothing to fear. I have learned that it's easy to start feeling at home in the upper reaches of the unconscious –

we don't drown; we don't get lost.

If I do get scared at any point, I return to a simple, trusting, childlike spirituality. I ask my guardian angel to hold my hand. Or I simply say the Lord's Prayer. I find those ancient words, learned in early childhood, remarkably reassuring and protective.

I have found useful guidelines to the inner wisdom in a book that was published when Timmy turned three: *The Intuitive Healer* by Marcia Emery. She explains how to shift into an intuitive state through dreams and meditation.

On her advice, I have started taking more notice of my dreams, and those quick images that pop into your mind when you're falling asleep, or waking up, or just daydreaming.

People often say, "But I don't remember my dreams."

I can identify with this. I don't remember mine all of the time. I can go for weeks without remembering much of any value.

But then, sooner or later, I will want to look inside my dreams again for the insights they contain. And then I adopt the following technique that is helpful for opening all aspects of intuition: *notice what you notice*.

If I'm not remembering much, I start by consciously noticing what I do notice – however tiny and apparently insignificant. Even if I only remember a fragment of a dream, or even just a feeling that I wake up with, I register it. I write it down in a dream diary that I keep by my bed.

Over successive mornings, I find that I remember more and more from the previous night's dreams. As soon as I can, preferably before I've got out of bed, I write them down in as much detail as I can. I give each dream a title. Then I read them back like stories, but I don't force them to fit into theories. I just enjoy them and live with them.

One thing I quickly notice is that the feelings I experience in my dreams correspond exactly to feelings I have towards something in my waking life. For example, if I experience small, constricting situations in my dreams, these very likely reflect a constricting situation in real life. Conversely, wide, stunning views and broad avenues often tell me that in real life I'm moving in the right direction.

Over time, I find that I remember more dreams. I get more images that pop into my mind out of nowhere. And I receive useful inspirations to help me in my work.

At this point, I frequently encounter another problem: I'm remembering *too* many dreams and images. It can become overwhelming. So then I put away the dream diary, and only get it out for the big dreams, or when I especially want to know something.

If I am seeking the answer to something, I ask a clear question before I go to sleep. I may mull over the question briefly. Then I consciously hand my question over to deeper guidance. In doing this, I allow myself to be in a trusting, childlike state, handing over to a loving, compassionate presence who is bigger and wiser than me.

When I release my question in this way – and it's not always easy to do – I get useful answers. Sometimes an answer comes in straight away, in the form of words, or an image that may be symbolic. Sometimes it comes to me the next morning, with the memory of a very vivid dream. And sometimes I simply wake up, knowing the answer.

During our two years of childhood in Russia, my two siblings and I had a fairy tale book called *Vasilisa the Beautiful* that was popular at bedtime. Vasilisa, the heroine, was often helped by a little doll given to her by her dying mother. The mother told Vasilisa that if she needed help, she should give the doll a little to eat and a little to drink, and the doll would help her.

Vasilisa's doll contained all the protective love and wisdom of her mother. It was also the voice of inner guidance. When Vasilisa was in trouble, perhaps facing danger from the cannibal witch Baba Yaga, the doll would say, "Go to sleep, Vasilisa, for morning is the mother of counsel."

I love those words: "Morning is the mother of counsel." There's something so peaceful about them, and it's true. If we nourish our intuition on a daily basis, and allow ourselves to sleep and rest in the night, solutions do arrive with the clarity of morning.

If I find it hard to quieten my teeming thoughts, I take it as a sign that I need to spend more time peacefully, in meditation.

I think meditation works rather like a tonic. When I spend 20 minutes a day meditating, my mind becomes generally calmer and my whole life seems to follow suit. I simply sit still and focus on my breathing. Or I count my breaths, from one to four, and start again. Or I focus on a particular image in my mind, such as a flower, or a leaf.

Some people meditate at a regular time every day for years on end. I don't. Like most of my activities, I do it for a while, and then I stop, or perhaps do it less frequently. Then, sooner or later, I feel the need to start a regular practice of meditation again.

This general approach of meditation and dream work is deeply rewarding. It fills me to the brim with happiness. If I compare myself now with how I was in my 20s, I see that it has transformed the way I work. Instead of straining every day, like Sisyphus pushing his rock up the mountain, I am more likely to approach any mental task with a sense of ease.

I usually spend a little time simply tuning into the task, whatever it might be. I trust the ideas that pop spontaneously into my head, and go with them when they feel right.

Here is a small example of this approach in action. Recently I set out to redesign the letter heading of the Microcephaly Support Group. This friendly group of parents was recommended to me by Contact a Family, later to be known as Contact, which is a charity that provides invaluable help to families with disabled children. In the Microcephaly Support Group, our children all have one thing in common: their heads have not grown as much as the norm. Hence: microcephaly – 'small head'.

Not being a designer, I was planning simply to alter the font and arrange the words as well as I could on the page.

Suddenly, out of the blue, an image popped into my head. This image was a smiley face – with a difference. An invisible hand started at the top of the face. A pen stroke went down, around and up again to draw the head shape. But the beginning and end of the circle did not meet. Instead, they overlapped. The resulting face was smaller at the top than it would normally be, and the overlapping pen strokes at the top looked like two tufts of hair.

The invisible hand then gave the face two eyes, a suggestion of a nose, and a smiley mouth. The face looked happy and friendly. However, because the circle hadn't closed properly, the forehead was more compressed than it would conventionally be.

Straight away, I knew it would make a great logo for the Microcephaly Support Group. Nothing else could so accurately show what microcephaly is about. Our children might have developed completely conventionally, if it weren't for one devastating fact: their brains did not grow as large as most people's.

I also really liked the happiness of the image. Our children with microcephaly are often gorgeous, with lovely personalities and a great capacity for happiness. Being a parent of a child with microcephaly isn't all bad – quite the opposite – and the image reminds us of this.

Later that day, I walked up to Cedars Health Club on Richmond Hill for a swim. I picked up a locker key at reception, went to the changing room and there, on my locker door, I found a little sticker with a yellow smiley face grinning at me. It wasn't the sort of thing you normally found in that well-kept place. Perhaps a child had put it there.

The tiny coincidence was startling.

At the same time, seeing that smiley face made me feel that I really was on track with my idea for the logo for the Microcephaly Support Group.

I find that's how it works. When I start tuning into my unconscious, through tools such as meditation and dreams, I come across many coincidences, and serendipitous things that just seem to happen out of the blue. After a while, it begins to seem increasingly normal.

It's also worth noting that I was feeling happy and relaxed when I went to Cedars Health Club. It's a lovely place, with a towering cedar tree by the entrance, and an aromatherapy-scented air of well-being.

When I am happy, serendipitous coincidences become more common. It's as if I am in the flow, and the universe gives me signs along the way that I am flowing in the right direction. My creativity also increases along with my intuitive abilities. Things get better and better.

When I am unhappy or tired, which often amount to the same thing, the coincidences dry up. Instead I have a sense that there is no clear way forward. Any signs that I see are accurate reflections of my fearful state of mind. Things get worse and worse.

The only thing that can really change my state from unhappiness to happiness is my own decision to change my mindset. It's as if there is a binary switch deep inside me. I can switch it on, meaning I am open to life, or I can switch it off, meaning that I am closed to life.

If I make a conscious effort to switch the binary switch on, flow starts once more.

Once I recognise this fact, the choice becomes a no-brainer. I choose... life.

Signs from the unconscious

About five months after Timmy's christening, Tessa faxed me

a quotation, which is I think fairly well known. Tessa's version was attributed to Goethe. However, several days after she sent it, I came by chance across the same quotation in a book, only this time it was attributed to a Scottish mountaineer, William Hutchinson Murray, who climbed Everest in 1951:

Concerning all acts of initiative (and creation), there is one elementary truth, the ignorance of which kills countless ideas and splendid plans; that the moment one definitely commits oneself, then Providence moves too. All sorts of things occur to help one that would never otherwise have occurred. A whole stream of events issue from the decision, raising in one's favour all manner of unforeseen incidents and meetings and material assistance which no man could have dreamed would have come his way.

The Swiss psychologist Carl Jung called this kind of meaningful coincidence "synchronicity", a lovely scientific-sounding word that doesn't disguise the fact it's a deeply strange process, beyond our conscious reckoning.

Despite its strangeness, we do, most of us, accept coincidence as an almost homely factor in our lives. Those telepathic moments when you and a friend or relative think the same thing, or buy the same item of clothing, or plan to ring each other on the same day, are all natural, everyday activities for the unconscious realms of our mind.

In the realm of the unconscious, there's nothing inexplicable about coincidences at all, because the unconscious – as Carl Jung realised – is actually a collective thing.

At first I found this baffling – how on earth can we all share the same unconscious mind?

But then, rather neatly, my unconscious helped me. Into my mind popped an image of the house in which I am writing.

There is something unusual about this house. It harbours a secret, up in the attic.

Our little house is one of a terrace of houses in Richmond, Surrey. The entire terrace was built out of London brick in Victorian times. When we moved in, we were amazed to discover that the loft space above us was effectively just a long tunnel under the rafters. It would originally have run along the whole length of the terrace.

Here and there, house owners had started to build dividing walls to turn their section of the collective loft into a private space. During the time we have lived here, more dividing walls have been built. We ourselves have joined the dividing frenzy and separated our loft space from the others.

I think the loft space as it used to be, before all we gentrifiers got hold of it, is a good analogy for the human psyche. We humans tend to act as though we are separate: unique islands of consciousness. We may think that no one can read our thoughts. But an essential part of our psyche has no dividing walls. That essential part is our unconscious. Through our unconscious we are linked to everyone.

The analogy may not be exact. Our loft space is small and cramped compared with the other rooms in the house. My unconscious, in contrast, feels much bigger in relation to other parts of my brain. My unconscious also doesn't feel as though it exists in a space 'upstairs'. It feels as though it lies simultaneously beyond, within and behind everything I consciously know. It stretches out in all directions, and also in none at all. It is truly everywhere.

However, I don't really know where my individual unconscious finishes and the collective unconscious, as Jung described it, begins. I wonder if the boundaries are indeterminate, like an estuary meeting the sea. All I know for sure is that our collective unconscious is vast, truly vast. It might even be described as infinite. At the same time, I wonder if it might sit comfortably on the tip of a pin.

It seems to me highly possible that the unconscious occupies a realm where the normal units of measurement simply do not apply.

The implications of that thought are astonishing. It means we have access, potentially, to all knowledge.

The process of extracting this knowledge is not like reading a book. Although solutions may pop into your mind instantaneously, you can't *make* this happen. There is an essential aspect to the equation that requires us to be passive. We ask a question – that's the important active part – and then we allow ourselves to be a receptive space in which the answer will emerge.

I think there are many techniques to help us do this effectively. The following example is how I like to do it at the moment, although over time I notice that my methods vary.

I concentrate on my breath, going in and out. Or I focus mentally on an imagined item. A favourite one of mine lately has been tiny spore capsules, shaped rather like a grain of wild rice, but much smaller, on spindly red stalks above the vivid green cushion of moss on our garden wall. Other times, I imagine a leaf in all its intricacy. Or I might look out of my window and see the green leaves fluttering on a tree, a living lace against the blue sky beyond. I like to lose myself in watching the pattern of fluttering green and blue.

Or maybe I watch a candle flame.

Focusing on one small thing is a great way of connecting with infinity, because infinity is contained in every small thing.

As I concentrate, I think about my question. I put my question into words, trying to be as clear as possible.

Frequently, a moving image pops into my mind. It's like watching a movie on an internal screen. In my case, the movie is generally silent.

Sometimes I don't see a movie at all. Instead, my mind becomes a radio receiver, and I hear a short phrase or even a single word. It's as if there is an internal voice.

Sometimes, being human, nothing whatsoever happens, and I am left feeling puzzled.

So then I just accept that the answer may well flash into my mind later at a point when I've truly let go of trying to get a 'result'. It might arrive in a dream that night. Or I might even realise that the answer is sitting inside me.

As a general rule, the more I let go of attachment to outcome, the more likely I am to receive an answer. However, if I *am* attached to the outcome, I can still notice signs that seem to shine out and speak to me.

One thing I've discovered is that my own mindset can make a big difference to the answers I get. If I am fearful in any way, I tune into fearful answers. So I try to avoid that. Fearful answers are no help to anyone.

Basically, what I put into the unconscious is as important as what I take out. There's something hugely and accurately reflective about it.

If I send horrible thoughts to somebody else, for example, these horrible thoughts have a nasty habit of coming back to me in some form or another. I end up having a really bad day.

So if I do find myself thinking horrible thoughts about somebody else, I try to remember the trick of opposites. Instead of cursing them, I mentally send them a blessing. I was taught how to do this very recently over a series of dreams which I call my Unconditional Blessing Dreams, part of a 'night tuition' course that came to me while I slept. In one dream, I was shown countless numbers of murderers. They weren't trying to murder me. They had murdered people in real life and now were in some sort of limbo.

It was horrific. I was desperate to get away, but the murderers and I stayed motionless, as though in a tableau.

Eventually, something caused me to change my feelings towards the murderers. I began to feel compassion. I sent them unconditional love and blessing. I forgave them. Instantly, all the murderers simply vanished.

In another dream I was shown people who were deceitful – habitual liars. Again, I didn't want to be with them. I tried to get away but couldn't. Again, I eventually felt compassion for them. I sent them unconditional love and blessing. I forgave them. And again, instantly, they vanished.

In yet another dream I was shown thin-lipped people from the past, mainly women, who were the epitome of pained duty, stripped of spontaneity and joy. Fairly quickly this time, I sent them love and blessing, and they vanished.

The message was clear: when faced with difficult people, send them unconditional love and blessing. They will either disappear, or the problems will diminish.

Of course, Jung would say that all these characters were aspects of the dreamer's own self – my shadow self. I can go along with that. So in sending love and blessings to those troubled dream characters, I also sent love and blessing to previously unloved aspects of myself.

Unconditional love and blessing

Loving the parts of yourself that you are not proud of is good work. It is transformative. Can you look into a mirror and say, "I love you"? How does that make you feel?

I have learned how to feel unconditional love and blessing towards another being – any other being, including myself.

Timmy has been the best teacher of all in this respect. I'm writing these paragraphs late at night. Earlier, I tucked him into his bed. He put his arms around me and I relaxed into his hug. As always, I felt the calm, uncluttered, loving energy that is so much his signature. Although he can get cross, there is no spikiness to him. He doesn't judge us. That makes him so relaxing to be with. His lack of judgement somehow enables me to be more truly myself. Because of his attitude, I am not trying to distort myself in order to please him... and then resenting that distortion, because it necessitates my becoming less authentic.

I know our son truly loves us just as we are. That is so liberating. That is the experience of heaven on earth. Ironically, although he needs us to help him function in this physical world, he is not emotionally needy. He is not demanding in the slightest. It's as if he knows he is fully, divinely loved, just as he is.

In the field of unconditional love, Timmy has been the teacher, and I have been the student. It has been relatively easy for me to feel unconditional love towards someone like him who feels it towards me. It is harder to feel love towards someone who is looking at me critically. It is impossible when I am looking at others critically. But I am now working on it.

Quietly wish others well

There is a meditative exercise that I like to do. It helps me to see all humanity with an open heart. When I first began the exercise, I found it difficult. But the more I have practised it, the easier it has become. I call it the Poppy Exercise, because the first time I did it, I imagined standing in a poppy field – a favourite place next to my grandparents' cottage that I used to visit as a child. In the meditation, every poppy represents a human being. Seeing people as poppies makes it easier for me. It's as if I am able to see through a person's worldly identity, through to their soul beyond.

You can find the Poppy Exercise in the Appendix at the back of this book. Do try it if you are drawn to. It can be tremendously helpful.

'Difficult' people do still pop up in my life of course. We all encounter difficult people. However, for me this has become a rarer event than it used to be. When I do meet someone difficult, this is what I do. I don't always remember at first – I get caught up in the drama of disliking someone. But sooner or later I remember, and I am always grateful for the following strategy.

First of all, I silently acknowledge that the other person and I have our differences, but nevertheless I send them unconditional love and blessing. I silently wish them well. I wish that they may truly thrive. And then I let them go. I let all attachment to outcome go.

More times than I can tell you, the problem disappears. Either the person somehow becomes much easier, or they seem to disappear from my life, though never in a nasty way. This is kindly work.

Messages from my disabled self

So how does all this relate to children with disabilities? I believe the collective unconscious means that we're all connected – we are all one, while also seeing ourselves as separate.

If I personally don't know how to deal with people who have disabling conditions, I also don't know how to deal with aspects in myself that are disabled. I am walling up part of my own psyche. The part of me that is mute or cannot walk becomes walled up. I am also highly likely to deny that any part of me is mute or cannot walk. "I am able!" I cry out. "It's somebody else who is disabled, not *me*."

I never approach the walled-up aspect of myself. I don't talk to her, or hug her. I don't acknowledge her. I may well forget that she is there – like a relative with learning disabilities who is kept at home rather than embarrass the rest of the family in public. Sadly, this happens more than we realise. It was the norm in our society once, and is still the norm in a number of societies around the world.

Unfortunately, because I choose not to accept the mute, disabled part of me, I simply don't realise that after she became walled up, she didn't have a chance to develop properly. She is like a scary relative that I daren't let out.

And yet, curiously, I never ask *why* a part of myself became mute, or unable to walk. What trauma caused this event? Was it one major event or, more likely, a whole series of traumas of varying degrees? Was it due to swingeing social conditioning that caused the wild, instinctive, natural part of me to feel discredited and shamed? Was there systematic devaluing of who I truly was? Was I praised for being good, hard-working and conformist? Was unkindness shown to my young self when I chose not to conform? And did I learn to join in with this process by walling up the aspects of me that I perceived as bad or undesirable?

If I did, I am not alone. Jung spoke a lot about the shadow self, those aspects of ourselves that are disowned as we grow up. It's an essential part of living within our own particular culture. By the time we reach seven, a major part of our shadow self has been formed. However, it can be added to throughout our lives.

The shadow self is often feared, because it can be an anarchic force within us, and within our society. However, there is no need to fear something that is actually part of who we are. My shadow self is less likely to be an undercover saboteur if I listen to her and respect her. Jung also said that the shadow self was a rich source of our creativity. It's full of valuable qualities that can help us lead happy and optimal lives.

I grew up doing well at school. I was intellectually able. I lived in the realm of achievement. The parts of me who didn't or couldn't go along with this approach to life didn't get a look in – until our son was born. Witnessing the disabled parts of myself as reflected in our son has been a profound and heart-opening experience.

Prayer is about receiving

There is an incredible tool of the unconscious that I would like to mention here: the power of prayer.

It took me many years to understand fully that prayer doesn't belong to a particular religion. There is no hierarchy in prayer. There is no need for a 'middle man' in a cleric's collar (although

I accept that many find regular churchgoing life-enhancing in myriad ways).

The vision of bliss I experienced in the year before Timmy was born showed me that we all have a direct connection with God – that we are all beautiful manifestations of the divine. Prayer belongs to everyone, and we can pray wherever and whenever we like.

My relationship with prayer has become transformed since becoming a mother. When Timmy was first born, and when he was going through painful tests and illnesses, I prayed frequently. Usually my prayers took the form of supplication: "Please can our son be safe and well."

However, at that time I was so fearful for Timmy that I couldn't allow the space within myself to hear the answers to my prayers. Praying became, for a while, an empty, hungering activity. I was operating at a frequency of desperation, and desperation became my world.

Gradually, only half-realising what I was doing, I began to add appreciation and thanksgiving to my prayer mix. The practice of prayer became a form of meditation. My dreams helped me to move in this direction. I received gentle pointers that suggested, whatever the situation, I always had a choice between fear… and love.

When my prayer became more thankful and appreciative, everything changed.

My understanding of appreciation is this: through appreciation, which traditionally might be called worship, I allow myself to be open to the divine: to witness it, to love it.

Appreciation might be as simple as stopping to look at a beautiful sky, or a tiny detail in a leaf or a flower.

Appreciation is about allowing the drawbridge of my individual psyche to be lowered and allowing the divine in all its shining wonder to flow freely through me. There is a sense of *yielding* to the divine.

My understanding of thanksgiving is this: it's about feeling gratitude for the many great things in my life, from the basic necessities like air and food and shelter, to the life-enhancers like friendship, love, laughter and beauty. There is a sense of *receiving* from the divine.

Appreciation and thanksgiving combined are, for me, about understanding and loving the infinite force of love and compassion that lies behind this movie of life. It's about allowing myself to be as a child: to trust the higher power that I have witnessed. To bathe in its love, and to receive the many gifts from it that come flowing as fast as I think of them.

I noticed that when I consciously began to appreciate all that was good in my life, there seemed to be more and more to appreciate.

There was nothing consistent about my changing outlook. I was still perfectly capable of waking up grumpy, or feeling wiped out after a medical appointment – but there were more good times. There was more *happiness*.

I began to believe that happiness is the cure for most known ills. I noticed that when our household was happy, the people in it tended to thrive.

Only when I added appreciation and thanksgiving to the mix did prayer become truly healing.

I am not a churchgoing Christian – there is too much that I am not drawn to.

However, I enjoy the wisdom that may be found within the Christian church, as it may in any church or temple.

I found a book that gave good principles for the therapeutic power of prayer: *His Healing Touch* by Michael Buckley. The author, who is a priest, suggests that you don't lay down a blueprint: after all, you can never know exactly what healing someone else requires.

Instead, if it's for your child, pray that your child, and you, be open to healing, and that the healing will reach your child and work on them in whatever ways they need.

I love the sense of 'letting go' when I do that. I am letting go of attachment to outcome.

It's important to understand that healing may not simply mean healing of physical ills. It may occur also, or instead, on a psychological level, bringing you peace.

Recently I have tried this at night with Timmy when he has started an illness, and his breathing has changed in the course of my prayer, and he's been fine the next day. This has happened several times. I don't understand how it works, but will certainly add it to my toolbox of well-being strategies.

As I metaphorically place it in there, I notice another strategy sitting next to it. Curiously, I take it out and study it. This is one that Steven has brought to the family. I see a small cardboard box, with Nepalese figures painted on it, a depiction of its contents. I breathe in a fragrance of incense, and catch the extreme freshness of snow in high places.

What should we call this strategy?

Let us call it... adventure.

10. Everest

There's a picture hanging at the bottom of our stairs that I like very much. It's a silhouette of mountain tops. The shapes are so simple, it's really just an abstract of blue, black and white: landscape pared down to the barest essentials. You can see three dark peaks, with deep blue sky and dots of fluffy clouds hanging neatly above.

You may also notice an aura of lighter sky, signifying sunrise, emanating from behind the black rock.

This is the roof of the world: the Himalayas. The central peak in the picture, by no means the most impressive from this angle, is Everest. Named in honour of a British surveyor general of India, 'Everest' is a surname that actually derives from the River Eure in France. Steven told me the indigenous names for the peak we call Everest, and they seem more fitting, with an awareness of the sacred wrapped into them. The Nepali name is 'Sagarmatha', meaning 'Head in Heaven'. There is a general sense of 'Mother of the Universe'. The Tibetan name is 'Qomolangma', or 'Peak of the Sacred Mother'.

Returning to 'Everest', I learned recently that the eponymous surveyor general pronounced his name, 'Eve rest'. This neatly brings us back to the idea of an archetypal mother of humanity, resting as she watches her creation unfold.

Steven took the photo himself. One morning, very early, he left his snug sleeping bag. He trudged up a mountain called Kala Pattar (or 'Black Rock'). When he reached the top, 18,500 feet above sea level, he waited there, in the dark and the cold, for dawn to light the sky. And then, with a mixture of awe, delight, numbness and euphoria, he saw the summit of Everest, and took his photo.

The thing is, it's not just a holiday snap of the world's highest mountain. It's a record of how one man, Timmy's father, learned how to cope with every parent's nightmare: caring for a painfully vulnerable child who would never score any of the goals that fathers tend to wish for.

Steven's way of coping was to travel to Everest and help raise thousands of pounds for sick children in the process.

It's interesting that we both became a lot happier when we stopped focusing on our own disadvantages, and started to use our skills and energies to help others. But reaching that point took time, and a lot of support from others.

Steven's journey began with a phone call. At the time he was personal finance editor at a national newspaper. His liking for hill-walking was well known among friends and colleagues.

The phone rang. He picked it up.

"Hello, Steven, Lewis here. Do you fancy going for a walk?"

"Sure," said Steven. "Where were you thinking of?"

"The Himalayas."

Lewis McNaught, managing director of Gartmore, was helping with the trip. His company was sponsoring it. The aim was to get the youngest British person to the top of Everest, and raise money for Great Ormond Street Hospital. There were four climbers in the team, all with a military background, all with an inspiring air of "We can do this". Neil Laughton, leader of the trip, was an ex-Royal Marine, a member of the SAS, and was shortly to become a successful businessman and motivational speaker. He had the rather unusual hobby of raising funds for Great Ormond Street by climbing the world's highest peaks – one from every continent.

Another climber was Geoffrey Stanford who would become, many years later, the headmaster of Fettes School in Edinburgh.

The other two climbers were childhood friends: Mick Crosthwaite, the slightly older of the two, would go on to become a successful businessman; Bear Grylls, then aged 22, was destined to become a world-famous adventurer, author, TV presenter and Chief Scout. But all that was a long way off.

Steven was one of the trekking members of the team. His role was to write up the expedition for his paper.

The training took months, although I was never clear exactly what it entailed. There were meetings in a number of London pubs and restaurants to discuss various aspects of the expedition. And there were regular visits to the gym.

The individual team members also had to raise sponsorship money. Steven did this by writing letters to every financial company he knew through his work. Banks, building societies and insurance companies gave him amounts ranging from £100 to £1,000. The sums quickly added up.

But it wasn't all about collecting cash. Steven turned out to be skilled at getting free equipment, flights and other supplies from sponsoring companies. Neil took to calling him "Mr Midas". Steven sourced quite a range of equipment, including clothing, clever tea bags that contained instant milk, computers and a coveted satellite phone – cutting-edge new technology at the time.

When I saw the growing evidence of Steven's acquisitions, I have to admit I did wonder if it was all strictly necessary.

"How many palmtops do you need in the Himalayas?" I asked cautiously, studying a tidy pile of digital devices. "They'll all be used," murmured Steven. He seemed abstracted. I looked closer. He was squeezing buttons on a watch I hadn't seen before.

"What's that?" I asked.

"My new Alti-Thermo Twin Sensor," he replied. "Do you know we're at exactly 189 feet above sea level here?"

He looked down again. "Ah, it depends on what pressure setting we're at. When you factor that in, it's nearer 100 to 110 feet...."

After that, I kept quiet. Steven, like many men, loves gadgets, and can justify anything on grounds of usefulness and good value. Why else, at the time of writing, do we currently have one laptop, three flight simulator programs, two joysticks and one throttle on our coffee table? (Answer to come in a later chapter.)

In between dinners and fundraising, climbers and trekkers went off for training sessions in the Lake District, Scotland, and Wales. Each time, Steven returned looking shattered but happy.

And then, just six weeks before departure, he returned with a sprained ankle.

"It'll be fine," he kept saying anxiously. "You'll see... Do you think it will be fine? Six weeks should be long enough, shouldn't it?"

One Sunday just before they left, some members of the team convened at the top of an office block in the City of London and abseiled off. A television crew filmed them. Timmy and I went along and soaked up the sunshine on the roof while daring people, one by one, hooked themselves on to a rope and slid over the side into thin air. Timmy enjoyed watching the action. He was intrigued to see his dad, among many others, disappear over the edge. Then, later, one by one, they would appear again on the roof. It was a spectacular, open-air version of 'Now you see me, now you don't'. There was an adventurous social buzz, and he lapped it all up.

The watchers were invited to have a go, and quite a number did.

I was not tempted. I feel uncomfortable around heights. Specifically, I have a fear of standing high up, next to an abyss. Height in itself doesn't worry me. I'm happy enough to be in a plane, up in the sky. In my dreams I often fly, and I love the dream-sensation of floating above the ground. In previous years, before we became parents, Steven and I used to go scuba diving around the coast of Britain. The sensation was one of flying like Superman, as we finned underwater over deep gullies and drops in the seabed. There was one magical, almost-but-not-quite-scary time, off the Farne Islands, where a seal came up to us under the water and tugged at our fins with his teeth, like a dog tugging at a stick in your hands. It was a memorable sensation.

But there's something about standing on a hard surface, near the edge of a sheer drop, that just makes my insides jump. Deep down, I think part of me believes that I *can* fly. Therefore, I do not fully trust myself to stay put. What if I just launched myself off, believing that I would be safe?

On the office block, while the abseiling was taking place, no one mentioned that the youngest spectator, Timmy, was a Great Ormond Street baby.

Although he personally hadn't had a great experience there, we were still aware that the hospital had a good reputation. It was a good cause to support.

In March 1998, three weeks after Timmy's christening, Steven and the rest of the team set off.

"Will you miss him?" was a question I was asked countless times.

"Of course not," I answered. I was still a fairly singular person. I genuinely didn't think I would. I imagined it would be fun, and we'd be communicating by satellite phone and email, so we'd be in touch nearly every day.

But the satellite phone blew up at Everest Base Camp. We only managed to speak twice more during the three weeks before Steven returned to Kathmandu. The silence was unnerving, even miserable. I hadn't realised how much I valued talking to him.

It seemed to me, emotionally, as though I were in a white-out. I had temporarily lost a source of reference that I'd taken for granted, until I was suddenly deprived of it.

I had to make do with imagining the trip from the itinerary and notes that Steven had left. And he filled in the gaps, vividly, on his return.

As a trekking member of the team, Steven's destination was Everest Base Camp. Although this was described as basically a stroll, it still sounded adventurous to me. There are narrow paths and rope bridges over gorges. If Steven was unlucky he might encounter yaks moving in the opposite direction. They don't stop for anyone.

The rope bridges in particular didn't sound like fun. They have wooden planks for floors, but lots of the planks are loose, and others are missing. I could picture Steven deciding which planks would be safe to stand on, while the whole bridge swung wildly over a deep ravine. Just thinking about it made my stomach jump.

I knew that every day while Steven walked upwards, he would be finding it harder to breathe in the thin air. His body would be adapting, in the amazing way that bodies do: new red blood cells would be formed to help transport the sparse oxygen more efficiently around his circulatory system. But then the next day he would go higher, and his body would have to adapt to even less oxygen....

Sometimes people don't adapt. They get headaches and then get very ill. There's no telling who will adapt and who won't. Drinking lots of water is meant to help. But even so, you can't tell.

At night, Steven would rest in a succession of simple lodges along the way. The air in these lodges was cold, very cold, despite the yak dung and kerosene burners that seemed to generate more odour than heat.

Sleeping quarters were basic. Steven could be sharing a thin wooden platform with several other trekkers. A proportion of these would snore. At least one trekker with insomnia would probably complain about the noise. The insomniac trekker might even grab the nearest trekking pole and prod the nearest noisy sleeper until they woke, swearing in any one of quite a few languages.

And if Steven wanted to go to the toilet in the night... well, he wouldn't. The toilet would be outdoors: a freezing platform suspended a few feet above the ground, with a hole carved in the middle. Below, a growing pyramid of urine and faeces would be frozen solid until one day it would be chipped away by the locals and carried down to pastures in the foothills where it would be spread as fertiliser.

But Steven would need to pee at night, because he was drinking lots of water to help him to acclimatise. So he would simply reach for his personal pee bottle, which he kept close by. All the trekkers did the same thing.

A pee bottle is similar to, but never to be confused with, a water bottle. Filling one by moonlight was, so Steven told me later, a whole new skill.

(I wonder if trekkers become psychologically attached to their pee bottles? On his return, Steven kept his by our bed for two whole weeks. It wasn't used. It just sat there on the floor, like a portly little statue to the god of micturition. I found this slightly unnerving. But I said nothing, though I was very tempted, and one day the pee bottle thankfully vanished.)

As the trekking team moved higher, they entered a strange, monochrome world. The photos Steven brought back show unreal landscapes of snow and shadow, stripped of colour except a deep blue sky. The images are spectacular. Among my favourites is a valley with dizzyingly high mountains grouped around like wise elders, their peaks trailing plumes of cloud into the deep blue heavens.

Although I am not tempted to do this strenuous trek myself, I like to gaze at that photo and imagine what it would be like to be there. Not in body, cold and aching, but in spirit, curious and open. I picture myself walking into the centre of that circle of peaked mountains. I sense their energy. The high winds bring them knowledge of the wider world. Their roots connect them with the planet's most ancient past.

The wise old mountain elders have witnessed civilisations come and go. What do they think of us? What advice might they impart to us?

What do they invite us to release to the winds... who do they invite us to become?

And what, beside stone, endures?

At base camp, every member of the team took part in a Puja ceremony. A Lama blessed every person, and every item of climbing equipment. This went on for several hours. It was an important part of the expedition: a spiritual pause that spoke of the very real danger that lay beyond this point.

No Sherpa guide will go beyond base camp without the Puja ceremony.

The Puja ceremony reminded me of the spiritual dimension that accompanies any difficult quest.

It's easy to see the act of climbing a mountain as a metaphor for surmounting one's own personal challenges. In which case, walking some way up the world's highest mountain becomes a really good metaphor.

The mountain in one's life can take many different forms – it doesn't have to be built out of granite. A major illness or disability is a psychological mountain. For Timmy, and countless other disabled children, every day can physically be hard work. Every day can feel like climbing a mountain. To do this, as he does, with a smile, is heroic.

Steven explored the hazardous icefall just above the base camp, and came back with increased respect for the climbers. He also realised on a deeper level that he did not have to reach every mountain peak. It's not always about the destination. It is always about the journey.

Steven and the other trekkers began the return descent while the mountaineers were still preparing for the summit. Two climbers in the team would eventually make it to the top: Neil Laughton and Bear Grylls. Each of them would progress to other remarkable adventures in the future. They would tell their own stories in time. And I think it's fair to say that every member of the expedition, climbers and trekkers alike, were altered in beneficial ways by their experience.

Meanwhile, Steven was glad to walk down. He loved the way

the air seemed rich and full of oxygen. He was full of energy. It was easy, easy.

When Steven returned, he seemed indefinably different. "It's given me more confidence – and more humility," was how he explained it to me. He started looking at everything differently. His job no longer seemed so satisfying. In the long term, he didn't really know where he was heading. In the short term, he needed a new challenge.

Steven told me about a motivating conversation Neil had shared with the trekkers on Everest, before they actually reached their own highest point. "Look beyond this summit," Neil said. "What is your next challenge?"

A year earlier, I had given Steven a flying lesson at Shoreham Airport, as a birthday present. It had been his first experience in a small plane, and he had loved it.

"I'm going to learn to fly," he told Neil and the others.

So as soon as he returned, Steven booked some flying lessons. At the time of writing, in 1999, he's gone solo and is well on his way to qualifying.

Where will Steven's licence lead him? Where will it lead us as a family? I don't know, but I can detect the unmistakable scent of adventure. It's an incredible gift to bring into our household: a feeling that anything is possible.

Anything is possible.

Timmy and I each received gifts from the Everest trip. Steven gave me a teal-blue pashmina shawl that is soft and perfect for meditating in. Timmy received a family of miniature Nepalese figures tucked into a cardboard box, and a sky-blue T-shirt with three golden embroidered yaks and the words "yak yak yak" above them. With his fair hair and blue eyes, he did look cute wearing it.

Also, in his room there is now a panoramic poster of the Himalayas, the 'roof of the world', which is a great thing for any small child to look up to and dream about.

11. Butterflies

Towards the end of Timmy's third summer, he got a bad ear infection. It went, finally, after two courses of antibiotics. But after that, he just wasn't wholly well. His appetite was poor, and nothing we tried seemed to shake him back into health.

One night in early October, I had a very unpleasant dream. I looked down and in the crook of my left arm, in my elbow, there were two flaps of blood. They looked like the wings of a butterfly, but they were two thin bags of blood. They were horrible. I hated them.

In my dream I was with a group of people. We were on some sort of guided adventure holiday. The leader, a mountaineer, took me to hospital. I knew this was the right thing to do, and that it would be all right.

But when I woke the next morning, I had a strong sense of foreboding.

I worried about our son. I started giving him an iron tonic, because I thought he might be low in iron, and it might perk him up. I was influenced by the dream, with its thin bags of blood.

One evening, as I was measuring a dose out, Timmy looked at what I was doing and said, forming the words carefully, with some difficulty, like a person unaccustomed to speaking (which he was – words were still few and far between): "I could die."

He said it conversationally, without any drama. It shook me. I wondered, as I always did when he came out with a phrase or a short sentence, what the chances were of that happening through random sounds, or whether he had actually said what I'd heard.

Maybe I should have taken him to the GP at that point and asked for a blood test. It's easy to say that with hindsight. I must have thought about it. But I didn't do it. I guess I was trying to protect him from yet more tests. And he didn't seem ill, just quiet. It was the sort of quietness that people get when they are convalescing from a previous illness.

Two weeks later, in mid-October, he suddenly got very ill in the space of a few hours. I took him to the GP first. The GP rang Kingston Hospital. Timmy and I went home and then we caught a cab to the hospital.

During the journey he was getting worse: very breathless, very pale and yellow. I was becoming frightened. Then, at the hospital, there was the inevitable wait to be seen. He got worse and worse. I asked for his oxygen levels to be checked, because I was terrified that he was short of air. But it was up in the mid-90s. It was okay.

But Timmy wasn't okay. He was far from okay. He was getting yellower and yellower. A registrar came and said, "He's very poorly." Blood was taken. By this time it was evening. Steven, who had been away on a work trip that day, got back and rushed to the hospital. He was with us when the registrar returned and said, "His blood levels are extremely low. He will need a transfusion."

The doctors said that our son had pneumonia and acute anaemia. He was admitted to the children's ward. There, the nurses asked us whether he slept in a bed or cot at home.

I said, "In a cot, but he comes into our bed with us when he's ill."

The nurses gave him a bed so I could sleep with him. I thought that was brilliant. When he had pneumonia at his previous hospital, I'd felt that he was isolated in his cot. I was sure that cuddles were healing.

Timmy was given his first intravenous shot of antibiotics that evening, and a drip. A blood transfusion was scheduled for the next day.

He seemed to improve during the night. He slept calmly and deeply. His colour improved, although he was still pale. In the morning, he woke up, looked around, yelped and clung on to me with all four limbs, like a rather gangly koala bear.

He was terrified, and wouldn't let go. I'd brought along his favourite toy of the moment, Piglet, and also a lion hand puppet (Timmy didn't have one main 'cuddly', the way other young children do). I made them walk curiously all around the bed and climb the equipment. They were a bit cheeky with it. Timmy liked that.

A nurse came in to say that Steven was on the phone, so I got up to speak to him but Timmy shrieked and held on even more tightly. He would only let me go when the nurse volunteered to hold him in her arms.

During the day he continued to improve. He was taken off the drip. He drank a fair bit and ate a tiny amount. We were transferred to a room with eight beds in it – a sign that he was a little better.

Timmy's bed was in the corner by the door. Next to us was a five-month-old baby girl, who had never left hospital since she'd been born, apart from one short outing to her family home. The sight of this small baby touched me a great deal. She didn't move much. It wasn't even certain whether she could see. But she liked music: she moved her limbs when I wound up a musical toy, or when I played Classic FM on a little radio, quietly, near Tim's bed.

When the baby's mother came in for daily visits, I found myself trying to encourage her. I said that Timmy at five months had had lots of problems, but that he was progressing well.

The mother said, so sadly, "I hope things do get better. I don't think they could get any worse."

During that day, with no intervention beyond the inevitable blood tests, Timmy did seem to improve. That evening he was given a small blood transfusion. Afterwards, he slept, and the next day he woke up full of energy. Some relatives came to visit, and they were surprised to see him looking so well. For Steven and me, the cramping worry and fear were beginning to diminish.

On the second night, Timmy was scheduled to have his second dose of blood. Two tiny bags of blood were hung up on a stand beside his bed. I looked at them with an unwelcome sense of recognition – my stomach jolted. They reminded me of the two bags of blood that looked like butterfly wings in my dream. In the end, though, these bags of blood were not given to Timmy. It was considered that he was doing well enough without them.

The next day he had another blood test. This involved the usual struggle of finding a suitable vein. During the three days he had been in hospital, the medics had had problems finding veins for intravenous antibiotics, blood and so on. So far they'd used veins in his feet, and the crook of his right elbow.

On this occasion, they settled on the crook of his left elbow. Watching them I felt a sense of inevitability, as though I had foreseen this scene. It was just like my dream, only in real life it was our son's arm, not mine. The bags of blood we'd already seen. Now a small amount of blood was being taken for a test. They used a little plastic butterfly clip to regulate the blood flow. Seeing that 'completed' my dream. Somehow, I knew then that in real life this frightening episode was over.

Later, a nurse came to tell us the result: Timmy's blood count had nearly doubled. "We can't really explain such an increase," she said. "But children can do funny things like that."

So he was discharged and we went home that day.

It was an odd episode. Timmy had seemed to get ill so quickly, and he got better so quickly too. I was left wondering what it had all been about, and what lessons there were to be learned from it.

First, I thought about the hospital itself, which was still fairly new to us at this time. I had been impressed by the staff, who had a relaxed yet efficient attitude that seemed to work well. I had been impressed by the emphasis they placed on play. I also liked the way they banned white coats from the ward. In other hospitals we'd visited with Timmy, the staff routinely wore white coats.

The episode had also reminded me of an important fact: orthodox medicine can be brilliant when it comes to emergencies.

Then I thought about that little baby girl who lived in the bed next to Timmy's. She had made such an impression on me. I wished that I could help children like her, and also her parents.

Later, I told our friend Tessa about the episode, with the dream that seemed to act as an early warning system. Tessa pointed out that butterflies in dreams are often symbols of transformation. That idea resonated with me.

Then, soon afterwards, I had two significant dreams. Both in their different ways suggested to me that we were entering a new chapter.

First, I dreamed that all this time since Timmy's birth I had been living in the hospital, sleeping on a camp bed in the corridor. But now I was packing up my camp bed. It was time to leave the hospital, because Timmy's hospital days were now finally over and normal life could resume.

At the same time, overlaying this theme, was a strong sense that it was time to be creative at home.

The second dream was altogether more mysterious. I dreamed that we were outside the hospital, and there was a series of columns that reached up high into the sky. They were like ancient, elegant Greek columns. They had a timeless quality: they had always been there; they would always be there.

In the dream, there was a challenge going on. I had to jump from the top of one column, to the next, and the next. But each time the gap was wider, and the final gap was so wide I knew logically I could never make it. However, I also knew that I couldn't stop now. I had built up my momentum and I just had to carry on, or I'd fall anyway. So I was leaping over the final impossible gap, and something was carrying me. I knew I would make it.

When I woke, I felt that the dream had some kind of reality in the future, and I was quite excited about this, in a nervous sort of way. There was a tangible sense of change in the air. We were moving on, whatever that meant.

12. Fleeing the market

We are at one of our weekly gatherings with the small group of mothers I met and bonded with when our babies were about to be born. The other children, all noticeably bigger than Timmy, run wild. He watches, smiles a lot, and plays with the ones who briefly slow down.

The mums drink tea and chat. As always, I am simply happy to be there, in a group of supportive friends.

Julie asks how I'm getting on with my book writing. She adds that I should include an account of our recent family holiday to the island of St Lucia in the Caribbean, and the things people said about Timmy there.

I realise that Julie is right.

St Lucia was a blend of sunshine and challenge.

It's where I lost my nerve in the marketplace.

It's where Timmy, health-wise, turned an important corner.

It's also where we met a kind, wise lady, who called herself Grandma, and she gave us a cotton thread that is as good as any to tie up the ends of our story.

Not the ends of the whole story, of course. Who knows where the whole story will take us? But the first three years of Timmy's life seem to have been particularly significant.

During these past three years a lot of internal changes have taken place in Timmy, his father, and me. Every new baby has the potential to be a game-changer for their parents. Timmy, with his unusual array of health issues, has been a fiery catalyst that has completely altered the way I look at the world. More than that: he has altered me from the inside out.

So yes, St Lucia should be included. I finish my tea, say goodbye to our friends, head home with Timmy, and start writing....

We are on a plane, a Virgin 747, heading to St Lucia. It is December. I love flying, but I am quietly nervous. We have never taken Timmy abroad and I am still very worried about his health. He has only recently been in hospital with anaemia, and he's also recovering from a recent chest infection. He is clearly not yet thriving.

I have an awful image that I can't get out of my mind: our little son returning to Britain in a body bag. You can tell from this that I am full of trepidation.

A woman in the seat in front keeps turning around to look at us. Eventually, she talks. Immediately, I wish she hadn't.

"Have you taken him abroad before?" she asks. "You're very brave. They often have spasms, you know."

"Spasms?" I echo, blankly. Steven is deep in a newspaper, and I envy him his separation from this unwelcome conversation. Timmy, between us, is sitting upright, looking alert and happy. He is gazing at a random point in front of him, yet taking in much more with his peripheral vision. His body language tells me that he knows this is a special event. He feels rather important and special to be sitting in this very different place. The way he is holding himself upright is significant. If he were bored, or unstimulated, he would flop to one side. But right now, he is sitting upright, taking it all in.

After a while, he will tune out. He will gaze into space, chat incomprehensibly, and laugh silently. We say that he is in 'La La Land' when he does that. But for now, he is being alert and noticing everything, from the interesting noises of the engines starting up, to the neat rows of people, each with their own colourful, noisy emotions that blend and spread like waves through the long and unusual room in which we are sitting.

Timmy likes the engine noise. He likes sitting between Daddy and Mummy. He feels both safe and adventurous.

I look blankly at the brusque woman in front of us, waiting for her meaning to become clear. Her unattractive words –

"They often have spasms" – must refer to Timmy's special needs, but I'm honestly not sure. The truth is, I'm not used to anyone referring to Timmy's disability quite so bluntly. I have been used to meeting friendliness, kindness and tact. I am not generally made to feel awkward or different, except by health professionals....

"I'm a physiotherapist," says the woman, explaining. As she continues talking it becomes clear that her experience of two other children with a noticeably small head, or microcephaly, leads her to assume that Timmy is subject to fits.

"Oh, he doesn't have fits," I explain, pleased that I can say such a thing. And with that denial I am aware of a basic instinct in me: I am keen to dissociate our son from those who are more badly affected in one respect than him.

There can be a funny sort of hierarchy among families with vulnerable children. With the best will in the world, we can't help quietly comparing notes. I wrote about it in an article for parents recently: "You meet another parent of a disabled child, and get talking. If your child is more able than theirs, you may feel a bit embarrassed, not quite sure what to say. And if their child is more able than yours... well, you smile and act like you can deal with that. And then you go home and weep."

In this, we are connected with everyone else around us, who may have no direct experience themselves of children with disabilities. Faced with more severe – or even, simply, different – problems than ours, we feel privileged and normal, and even a little embarrassed by our good fortune.

So here we are, about to take off for St Lucia, and I am feeling distinctly put out. Can't we just escape and go on holiday like anyone else?

At the first opportunity, after a final false smile, I turn my gaze away from the physiotherapist and open a magazine. I glance at Timmy and am glad to notice that he is unmoved by the woman's unwelcome comments. As we take off, I relax. This is a favourite moment of mine. I love the sensation of letting go. I am being carried up into the sky by this amazing miracle of engineering. I love the freedom of it.

As the plane ascends, I studiously make sure I don't make eye contact with the woman again.

I do realise, though, that she didn't mean any harm. In a sense she was simply reflecting back to me my own anxiety about taking our son so far from home.

But I do mind her evident belief that she can make personal comments about Timmy, in front of him, without even saying, "Hi," to him.

The truth is, there is no escape. When your child has disabilities, it's a bit like being a famous person. People notice you. Often they just stare and look away. Sometimes they come up to you with a particular sort of smile, and chat as though they know you.

You always have to be an ambassador for your own special child, as well as for the mythological country of Special-Needsia. Either that, or you become defensive and prickly and people don't dare talk to you. Or, perhaps, you stay at home and don't go on holiday.

Halfway to St Lucia, above the vast Atlantic Ocean, I suddenly catch up with the leaping dream I had after Timmy came out of hospital.

In the dream, I reached a point where there was no going back. In real life, suspended high in the air, I am also, literally, at the point where there's no going back. We are now closer to our destination than our starting point. The only way to go is forwards.

But the dream had another symbolic level of meaning. The Greek columns spoke of an ancient, timeless architecture. In the dream, the columns were free-standing in an open landscape. They supported nothing, except air and ideas. They simply stretched upwards.

In the dream, I was leaping from the top of one column to the next, and the next, on a journey that felt risky yet also uplifting. And then I reached a momentum, where the only way to go was forwards.

The columns speak to me of a sense of order, fairness and an equal society. They speak to me of a plan – perhaps a life plan. I can't see the plan, but I catch glimpses of it from time to time.

At some point during the flight, I realise on a deeper level that my fear is not really about going on holiday. It's about going through life.

When we arrive in St Lucia, we walk out of the plane and down some steep steps. The air feels warm and humid, so different from the air that we left. I am carrying Timmy in my arms. I am aware of him turning his head to look at the plane as we leave it, but I can't see his expression, because I'm busy looking at the steps that I am gingerly descending.

Suddenly, he starts shaking violently in my arms. I feel the jerky movement, stop descending, and look at him, worried.

Then I realise: he's *laughing*. He is looking at the enormous plane and he is laughing. It dawns on me that when we boarded at Heathrow, we walked through a corridor directly into the plane. So Timmy didn't actually see what he was entering. Steven, just behind us, also notices Timmy's reaction. We look at each other and beam.

For Timmy, this is the first time he has seen what he's been sitting inside for the past eight hours. It must seem like magic to him – like the world's most amazing lift that has transported him from a cold place to a warm, lush one.

He looks happy and excited, glowing and dewy in the warm atmosphere.

We are driven through lush banana plantations with coconut trees looming over, through steep rainforest with tree ferns etching the sky. The air is so warm and humid. Timmy starts coughing. When we arrive at our hotel, he coughs up some hard, compacted greenish phlegm that looks... old.

We are surprised, but remember after his chest infection six weeks earlier, his consultant had mentioned that he could produce phlegm for a long time to come.

Timmy will continue to cough up old phlegm all through our two-week holiday. Over time, the phlegm will become looser and paler, until it will finally disappear. It is like one of his illnesses in reverse, but there are no other symptoms, and is somehow puzzling.

During this period, he is on a course of homeopathy, and I am also giving him daily skin brushing according to a programme set up by Kerry, his occupational therapist in England. He has also just had an osteopathy session. And he is absorbing the sunshine of St Lucia, and the warm, humid air.

Who knows which if any of these things is causing the changes in him, but they will lead, by the second week of our holiday, to a new appetite, and good health. This good health will stay with him over the following year, and he will gradually become stronger.

So, we know that something good is going on, but nobody in St Lucia is aware of this. What they see is, for them, a highly unusual child: blond, blue-eyed, impossibly long-limbed, and painfully thin.

In the hotel, the beautiful, graceful hotel staff are full of friendliness towards him and us. A member of the housekeeping staff brings him a flower or two every day: a hibiscus, a couple of roses. "I am Grandma," she tells him, and us.

When we travel around the island, people often stop short in their tracks to stare at him. Most of the women are kind. They say, "You are beautiful, you are so cute, what is your name?" But every day at least one person will add, "What is wrong with him?" Or, "Can he walk?" I feel like flinching every time someone asks these questions.

Sometimes, usually from men, we get advice: "You should feed him more."

As if we haven't tried!

A few say: "You should keep him here and let the sunshine of St Lucia cure him."

Some of the advice makes good old-fashioned sense: many women make sure we're not giving him ice-cold drinks or very cold food if he has a chill.

Other suggestions are a bit bold for our restrained British ways.

"You must stand up and claim healing for your child," admonishes a waitress. "Stand up and claim it from God!"

I wonder why we never see people in wheelchairs in the streets, but one day in Castries, the capital city, I realise why: there is no wheelchair access anywhere. The streets contain open drains.

In Castries we enter the crafts market, which appears to be mainly full of T-shirts with slogans. There are many aisles, and each seems to be full of more or less the same things. Steven walks off to video the stalls. I walk on slowly, pushing Timmy in his buggy, looking at the wares.

Then it happens.

A tall, stocky woman stares at me and says in a deep voice, "Is your child sick in de heart?"

For some reason this spooks me. It seems like voodoo. I know Timmy is not sick in de heart. We saw his heart on ultrasound in one of his many tests and were informed that he has a textbook, healthy heart. But saying such a thing... it seems like inviting trouble. I mumble something, and walk on. A few steps further, and a man asks, "Can your child walk?"

Everyone is staring. It is too much. I can't cope with this scrutiny. I walk rapidly out of the crafts market, pushing Timmy in his buggy before me, and then realise that I have to enter it again to find Steven.

Thankfully Steven is just inside the entrance. He is filming a T-shirt that says, "Same shit, different island."

"You shouldn't let it get to you," he says, unperturbed.

"I just don't know what to say to them," I reply.

"I don't think you noticed," continues Steven, snapping the video camera shut, "but there was a man at the entrance when we came in who asked me what was wrong with Timmy. I said, 'Nothing, what's wrong with you?' and walked on. Remember you can always choose what you say."

That final sentence comes from a disability article that I wrote recently. I feel abashed. Why has it just become so hard to follow my own advice? Perhaps it's the deluge of interest that has thrown me. But all this is just another obstacle, which I can learn how to overcome.

"Can he walk?" asks an assistant in a clothes shop the next day. "Why do you ask?" I answer, at last. 'Why' is such a little word, yet so powerful. It's a terrifically helpful starting point when it comes to standing my ground and reasserting myself.

"His legs are so thin," is the reply.

I answer that his legs are strong. He can stand with support. He can take steps holding on to furniture or people.

And then I ask the assistant what happens to children and adults on the island who cannot walk. I'm still wondering why we never see any in the streets.

"They stay with their families; that's what people want," she replies. And then she tells me about a friend's daughter who has similar problems. She's very concerned about her.

I walk out of the shop much happier. By asking, "Why?" I turned a question into a conversation, in which we connected and I learned something.

One evening at the hotel, I go out to the poolside table where Steven and Timmy are already sitting. They are looking up at the night sky. Timmy is pointing heavenwards.

"Dar," he says, pointing.

"Where are the stars, Timmy?" asks Steven. Timmy's finger points upwards again. "Dar," he says happily. They are both grinning. They think it's a great game.

What we don't know is that Timmy is going to have a thing about the stars – or perhaps, who knows, it's just a single star – for a long time to come. Sometimes he will say "star" perfectly. More often it'll be "dar". He'll love songs about stars, and pictures of stars. Many times, out shopping, he'll catch a stranger's eye, point upwards, and say, "Dar," and the clever ones will understand him.

And it all began in St Lucia, where his daddy taught him to look at the stars.

A few days on, in the south of the island, we follow a handwritten sign that says, "Mineral spring". We walk, following a local guide, along a narrow woodland path between breadfruit, papaya and cacao trees.

I am thrilled at this opportunity to walk among such gorgeously exotic plants.

The air is rich with a heady scent: woody, and smoky. It reminds me of the sandalwood oil that surrounded the mahouts like an aura, when we went to look for tigers by elephant in Bandhavgarh National Park, India, seven years before.

We were somewhat off the tourist trail there. We are also somewhat off it here. We know there is an official mineral spring nearby where tourists bathe in water that has been siphoned off, filtered, and put neatly in baths. We will visit that same sanitised spa ourselves, on our final day.

But today, we are doing it the unofficial way, the fun way. So we walk down into a gorge, following the narrow woodland path. Steven is carrying Timmy, who looks up and around, liking the trees.

As we walk, we hear a thunderous sound that gets louder as we approach: a waterfall.

I am enjoying this so much: it's a magical scene. The waterfall starts high up, and falls in a narrow cascade. The plunge pool has been lined roughly with concrete, with steps leading down into it. Though the concrete is not pretty, it is practical. We get changed. The guide, a local, is still nearby, so I change discreetly in a little hut with a mud floor and no door. Then Steven, Timmy and I step into the pool together.

The water is spa-warm. It is soft, and the strange heady scent hangs in the air above and around us. Timmy, in my arms now, is nervous and cries. The thunder of the waterfall is upsetting him.

I bob gently in the warm water and sway with him in my arms, soothing him, letting him float within my arms in the iron-rich warmth of it, like a baby in amniotic fluid.

As I soothe him, I also allow myself to be soothed.

Gradually, he relaxes. He looks around, wide-eyed.

After a while, I hand Timmy over to Steven and lie face upward in the water. I float, gazing up, up, up at the waterfall, up to the canopy of trees at the top of the gorge, up to the white sky beyond.

I am supremely relaxed, and happy.

The water is rich in minerals. It is supposed to be very good for the health. Whether this is true or not, I cannot say. But I do know that floating beneath thundering, falling warm water in (almost) undiscovered woodland is one of the nicest things I have ever done on holiday. For a little while I feel happy and relaxed, and that is all.

And I have heard it said that waterfalls, like butterflies, are symbols of transformation. Your life is like the journey of a raindrop. You begin in the heavens, coalescing into a drop of rain, falling to the earth, joining a stream that becomes a river. Maybe, as you journey downwards, deeper into your physical life, there is rough water, or even a sudden drop. One day you join the sea. You evaporate, and the process begins all over again.

This is what the river has been for me so far....

In the long, early stages of my journey I bobbed along, with small patches of turbulence at intervals along the way.

Then, gradually, I noticed that the water was flowing faster. There was a strange, unfamiliar sound ahead, becoming deeper and louder. Thunderous. I no longer felt safe....

And then it got worse, so much worse. I could no longer see land in front of me, just sky. It was as if the land was about to disappear, as if I was about to fall off the edge of the world. There was nothing I could do. I was helpless. Forces, far bigger than me, were sweeping me along.

And then... *whoosh!* There was no time even to scream. I was in free fall... plunging downwards in an unstoppable torrent of white water.

I was not in control. I was helplessly falling any which way.

All I could do was fall, fall, fall.

And then, like hitting a wall, I was in the plunge pool. I was bobbing up, then down again, and then up again.

I tasted the sweetness of life.

And then, scarcely stopping, I continued my journey, flowing where the river flows.

Today, the river and I are both at a deeper level. I have reached the next stage in my development and in my life. There will probably be many more adventures before I reach the flat, silvery calm of the estuary, if I make it that far. And then I will enter the sea.

But when I am an old, old being, I'll look back at the river of my life, and I will remember the time I went down a waterfall, and I will say, "That was when my life changed."

And curious although this may seem, I will remember that frightening, difficult time with fondness for what it brought me.

We fly back to England feeling very pleased with ourselves. Timmy has a slight, rather becoming tan. His hair has bleached white in the sun. He has a definite healthy glow about him. So do we. And we've proved something to ourselves: we can go on holiday; we can travel anywhere, the three of us.

Yes, we had to deal with some surprised looks and direct questions. But the answer to that really is simple. We will not hide at home. We will get out there and live life to the full. The more families who do that, the less surprising it will be to the rest of the world.

On our return flight we are carrying a small gift. It is from the beautiful St Lucian lady who called herself Grandma. The gift is special, because it belonged to her for many years, and she cared enough about Timmy to give it to us, three tourists on a fortnight's holiday in her country.

The gift is a book, slightly musty from life in a warm climate. Called *The Desire of Ages*, it seems to belong to a bygone era. It's a gentle study of the life of Jesus, complete with pencil lines around meaningful passages that have clearly been read, and loved over the years.

Between its pages lie two crushed roses, one red, and one white, which Grandma gave to Timmy. "Keep the petals, so he can remember," she said.

And then I remember what she said when we tried to arrange Timmy prettily in her arms for a photo. "It's okay, let him be himself," she said. So we did, and in the photo he looks relaxed and happy.

When I open Grandma's book, I can feel how well read it is, and how loved. She gave us her own personal copy, and that touches me.

There is something else that strikes me as significant: a blue thread that she used as a bookmark.

The blue thread is so like the sky-blue thread that I tied on to marble lace at the hermit's tomb in Fatehpur Sikri, in India. The two threads could have come from the same spool.

For me, the first thread opened this whole mysterious

business. And now it feels as though the second thread is closing it....

What do I mean by that? We are still living our story of disability. But we have moved on so far. We have moved from not coping, to coping. And in the process my heart has opened.

It's like this. The Indian thread was tied to a wish for happiness. The second thread comes within a book that refers to the human search for happiness.

On the first page it asks what people desire.

What would you answer? My answer would be something along the lines of happiness, love, good health and peace, for my loved ones, all living beings and myself.

Its pages are about the teachings of Christ: love yourself, love God, and love your fellow human beings. Be open to healing, and you will be healed.

The first thread I gave away. The second thread was given to us.

As I finger the blue thread from Grandma's book, I notice how my thoughts move beyond our small family circle to a wider community of disabled children and their parents. My personal therapy is, and always has been, to write. I wonder whether I will do more writing on this subject, and whether it will resonate with others too.

13. Remember your vows

Steven has taken Timmy to Covent Garden, to sit in Henry's Bar with a group of Steven's old college friends. The two boys will come back glowing from the fun of their outing. Steven will be full of stories of how Timmy sat sociably on Julie's lap and chatted, how he took Joanna's mobile phone and put it to his ear, saying, "Dad dad." How a drink of milk was ordered for him alongside the others' soft drinks. How at times he sat quietly in his own chair, playing happily while the others gossiped about last night's party.

You know: just normal stuff that small children do.

Later this evening Steven will say, pleased, "Timmy's really come on lately. He's become so… self-possessed. I really enjoyed going out with him. He was sociable with the others, and able to play on his own when he wasn't the centre of attention."

But I don't know this yet. I am sitting at my computer, writing a magazine article, and sneaking in a little book writing too. I am relishing the time and space on my own, loving the fact that Steven and his son can go out so easily.

For a long time, such activities were harder. We did them, but they were harder. Timmy would suffer from sensation overload. The noise would upset him. He would get tired. He wouldn't eat his supper. He would go to bed and very possibly develop a temperature.

We never took him out of Richmond without infant paracetamol.

As I write, in 1999, he can cope with and enjoy social groups just like anyone else. Although he still has significant developmental delays, and his body doesn't work for him as well as it might, he has lost a lot of the hypersensitivity that made outings so difficult for him. And while celebrating this fact, I have a very distinct, and growing feeling.

It's hard to put this feeling into words, let alone speak them out loud. But if I have to, these are the words I would choose: "What next?"

Teachings of Brian Duppa

Along The Vineyard in Richmond there is a row of elegant old dwellings. They're called Bishop Duppa's Almshouses. Above the ornate entrance gate is a stone tablet bearing this inscription:

I will pay the vows
which I made to God
in my trouble.

The words linger in my mind long after I've walked past them, pushing Timmy in his buggy before me. Each time we walk past, they have the same effect. There's a compelling honesty about the inscription. Bishop Duppa evidently didn't try to hide the fact that he went through hard times.

One day I look up Bishop Duppa, and this is what I discover. Bear with me, it's going to sound like a history lesson, but it's worth it.

Brian Duppa was born in Kent, in March 1589. His father was a brewer for the Royal Court, supplying beer to Queen Elizabeth I and her successors. Brian went to Westminster School as a King's scholar, and then on to the University of Oxford. There, in 1614, he gained a Master's Degree. After that, it sounds as though he travelled around Continental Europe for a while, as part of his continuing education. Within five years he was back in Oxford, where he was given the job of proctor, supervising the behaviour of the students. At the time of his appointment he was praised highly: "not only a most Excellent Scholar, but a Man of a very *Genteel Personage and Behaviour*." He was a good role model for others.

In due course, Brian Duppa took Holy Orders and became

an Anglican chaplain. Thanks to connections that his father had made in Court, and more that he himself had made at Oxford, he enjoyed a comfortable ecclesiastical career.

At the age of 37, Brian Duppa married a lady called Jane, who was older than him. It was a very happy marriage. They had no children, but a large, vibrant extended family between them. Many of the family members had Royalist leanings. Brian Duppa's career continued to flourish. He became bishop first of Chichester, then later of Salisbury.

Life was good.

Then, at the age of 48, something life-changing happened to Bishop Duppa, as he was now universally known. He was appointed tutor to the Prince of Wales; and quickly became a trusted friend and advisor to the prince's father, King Charles I.

But these were difficult times to become friendly with Royalty. Many in the country thought the King was too High Church, almost Catholic in his leanings, and that he was trying to impose these on a more Puritanical nation. There were warring factions in Scotland, Ireland and England. The fragile unity of the kingdom broke down, leading to Civil War.

When Charles I eventually lost his throne, Brian Duppa spent time with him in exile on the Isle of Wight, still tutoring the King's sons.

Eventually, King Charles was captured and brought to London. There, he was beheaded.

Brian and Jane Duppa retreated to live in Richmond, but they had very little money, as the ecclesiastical income was withdrawn. While Oliver Cromwell ruled Britain, the Duppas lived a quiet life, dependent on the financial support of friends. But he still worked behind the scenes to uphold the interests of the church he loved.

During a decade of Cromwellian rule, Bishop Duppa produced some beautiful religious writings. It was as if he went through a spiritual fire. When he emerged from it, he spoke and wrote from the heart and soul. Everything else was stripped away. Consider this prayer from *Holy rules and helps to devotion both in prayer and practice*:

> *Oh Heavenly Father, who hearest the prayers of all that seek Thee, purifie the intention of my Soul in all the prayers I make to Thee; that I may neither seek nor desire anything, but in relation to Thee.*

It's worth emphasising that he wrote those words during a bloody era when traitors were hanged, drawn and quartered. But it was also the dawn of the Age of Enlightenment. His writings reflect this combination of barbarism and transcendence. He understood the need not to get bogged down by worldly terrors, and the need to keep one's spiritual vibration high:

> *For overmuch solicitude and anxiety of Mind in worldly things, calls such a heap of Earth upon our Prayers, as will not suffer them to ascend.*

After ten years, Brian Duppa's old student, the Prince of Wales, gained the throne, becoming Charles II. The Duppas prospered once more, in a new and more democratic Britain. Brian became Bishop of Winchester.

King Charles II visited his old tutor on the dying man's 74th birthday. The monarch knelt to ask for the Bishop's blessing. On 26th March 1662, the day after the King's visit, Brian Duppa died. He was buried with honour at Westminster Abbey. Jane, his much-loved wife, survived him.

It is key to this story that as soon as he could afford to, Bishop Duppa gave financial help to others. He gave a substantial sum of money back to his community, to create almshouses – giving a roof to others who could not afford their own. And he wrote that honest and heartfelt declaration, for all to see, on the Richmond Almshouses: "I will pay the vows which I made to God in my trouble."

The original almshouses Duppa built were replaced in the 18th century. Today the 'modern' replacements look as elegant as any Oxbridge College.

There is something beautifully inspiring about Bishop Duppa's story. I like the fact that he supported his monarch even when it would have been politically expedient not to. I like the fact that during his Richmond years he worked quietly and tirelessly for the Church and for his parishioners. I love the purity of his spiritual writings. And I like that he wrote so honestly, revealing his feelings, in words that still exist on stone for all to see.

This is the crux of it: Brian Duppa believed in something, and stood up for his beliefs, openly and honestly, without being showy or indeed a martyr. He was able to be true to himself and those he loved in troubled times. He had the confidence and integrity to be a quiet but clear spokesman for his beliefs. He was uplifting and inspirational.

That is something to emulate.

Time to tell our story

By nature, I am not especially practical, or indeed political. I hold no position of power. And building houses is not my strength. But I do relate to the idea of being honest about our story. After all, what do any of us truly own, apart from our emotions and our experiences?

I believe that telling one's own true story can make a difference. Stories are medicine, for all who share them.

I would like to do my bit to help change attitudes towards children and adults with disabilities, simply by sharing our experiences. For me, that includes the inner world of emotions, insights and dreams. This account would not be an honest one if it were written in, for example, the external language of medicine or education.

The real, unvarnished truth is that parents of disabled children do not always cope, and the wider world hasn't really much idea of how to cope either. People think that anti-discrimination laws are enough, but these are just the first, primitive building bricks towards an integrated society in which disabled people are treated as the normal, equal human beings they are.

It's like this: the soft cement, that is spread like butter between building bricks and then hardens, is what keeps the bricks in place. A building cannot be erected without some kind of cement.

There is a corresponding social cement that helps to build a fair and equal society.

This social cement represents the way people think and feel. To put it simply, if people are able to love and accept themselves and all other members of their community, all members of that community will flourish.

This is not happening at the moment. There's just not enough acceptance around. We know, from our experience with our son, that there is ambivalence towards disabilities in our country. There is ambivalence about people who *look* different. There is ambivalence towards people who *behave* differently. This means that those who have cognitive and physical disabilities, and their families, feel segregated and isolated at least some of the time.

Of course many parents do cope, generally. But there is an awful lot of trauma along the way.

And sadly, so sadly, some parents do give up.

Earlier this week we learned of a little boy living locally, who has cognitive and physical disabilities, and epilepsy. He is just beginning to take steps, and he is apparently bright and watchful, although he doesn't talk.

Apart from the epilepsy, he sounds similar to Timmy. If anything, he sounds more mobile.

But there is a major difference.

His parents, middle-class professionals, are putting their son up for adoption. The process has begun.

I am so shocked and saddened by the news. It hits me in the solar plexus. It upsets me to my bones. It's the very last thing that Steven and I would ever choose to do. We just wouldn't do it, not ever.

Can you imagine having a child, and living with that child for several years... and then signing him away to strangers? I'm torn between bafflement and sadness. I find their decision particularly shocking, because their situation sounds so similar to ours.

Most parents of disabled children would never, ever want to give up their children. Many will tell you about the extraordinary love and closeness they enjoy with their child. That love sustains their children and helps them to grow up and bloom in their own unique and beautiful ways.

But we can be sure that every parent of a vulnerable child has suffered to a degree that they couldn't begin to put into words. They have most likely cried many, many times. Even if they haven't cried with physical, saltwater tears, they have cried on the inside, in a place that perhaps even they might not be able to reach.

Here is my truth.

I have cried after medical appointments, which are so often more brutal and painful for children than they need to be.

I have cried after thoughtless comments from others.

I have cried because I have had to see someone I love with my whole heart suffer in a wide variety of ways, day after day.

I have cried because my life has become restricted.

I have cried because I worry about our child's future.

I have cried because things were never meant to be like this.

My situation, and that of our son, has always felt worse when no one offers me hope... when no one says what I am feeling is normal... when no one says that our son is normal, that our small family of three is normal. When no one gives me a sense that I am a strong, powerful, wise person, who is doing a brilliant job.

I will remind you of something now. If you are living on this planet, you are normal. We are all normal. We are not the same: we come in different shapes and sizes. We have different strengths and weaknesses. But we are all normal.

Like all parents of a disabled child, I feel a lot better when other people simply accept Timmy, Steven and myself for who we are.

I don't, for the record, want someone I meet socially to say, "Oh, you're so brave, how do you cope?" I just want us to be treated as normal people.

I'd prefer not to be told, "I could never do what you do."

I'd rather not be asked, "What's wrong with him?"

And I particularly loathe the following variant: "Do they know what's wrong with him?"

Sometimes, if I'm feeling unhelpful, I will respond tersely, "Who are 'they'?"

That usually silences the enquirer. We both know that 'they' refers to doctors and other people in positions of authority. And we both know that if I am asking, I am not open to hearing such an answer. I am in the mood to *shred* such an answer. So the enquirer, if wise, stays silent.

And please, please save me from anyone who looks at Timmy or his parents with pity. It's infuriating. We are simply being ourselves. We are simply living our life. Our differences may be obvious, but everyone has differences. We all have challenges that we struggle with.

I would also rather that well-meaning health professionals did not assume that we'll meekly agree to whatever tests and treatment they choose to do. We'd rather that our views were listened to without a superior "I know better than you" smile.

Parents need to be given the confidence to listen to their own instincts. If you give up your instincts in favour of someone who believes he or she is an expert, mistakes will happen. Of course it's fine to consult the experts. But at the end of the day, instinct is the best guide any of us have. When your child is vulnerable, listening to your instincts may even be lifesaving.

Remembering those who didn't make it

In some cases, sadly, instinct may let you know that you have only a limited time together. If that is ever the case, as one bereaved father wrote recently to other parents in an Internet special needs support group, "Cuddle your child as often and whenever you can. Never hold back on the cuddles. Because afterwards, all you've got left are the memories of those cuddles."

I do know of several contemporaries of Timmy's who have not made it this far, who died of pneumonia during one of our long, damp, chilling winters. Pneumonia is one of the biggest killers of children under five. I have learnt to dread English winters, though I am working on liking them again. But for parents of vulnerable children today, it's almost as if we're still living in Victorian times.

I am going to tell you something sad now.

In Oldham last Christmas, I went with Steven and his aunt Norma to visit the grave of a kind and gentle uncle who died suddenly in November. Close by his grave was a sprinkling of children's graves. You could see immediately that they belonged to children, because they had soft toys and little Christmas presents on them. Some had little plastic windmills, spinning in the breeze.

I looked at the children's ages, marked on their headstones. Three, four, five... It was just too much. Tears welled up. I was face to face with the reality of young death, with the grief of parents as they placed toys on damp earth that should have been in warm, small, grasping hands. And those parents' grief will never vanish. They will have to face it day after day after day.

We walked with Norma deeper into the graveyard. We were looking for the grave of her second son, called Ian, who had died within days of being born. But there was no grave marked. "All the newborn babies were put into a single grave and there was no headstone," she explained. "That was the way it was done in those days."

Norma led us to a sunken area: just grass, with nothing on it. "It was here."

She must be one of the very few people who know.

At least we no longer put the children who didn't make it into unmarked mass graves, like tiny victims of a civil war. There has been some progress. But there is a way to go.

Paul's inspiring decision

This past week we've had Paul Donnelly, a delightful Irish friend, to stay with us. It's been his final week in London before he takes up a voluntary post in Uganda for two years. Paul is single, one of a large family spread throughout Ireland. He has given up his flat and his well-paid job, and has been saying lots of goodbyes over many pints of Guinness with an endless stream of friends.

His leaving party was last night. It was good fun. You can see that Paul's decision to give something back has gently shaken many of his friends. We all have the impulse in us, but it gets buried under the need to earn more, pay the mortgage, and look after our own family.

Something Paul said in his leaving speech struck a chord with me.

"A year ago I woke up one morning, and thought, 'Well, I have a good career, a comfortable flat, a lovely supportive family, great friends... there must be more to life than this.'"

In a way, that's how I feel. As Timmy's health improves I could just settle back into my comfortable life, and over time let the shaky past be gradually forgotten. But I can't do that. I've been in on the inside. Let me not kid myself: I am still in on the inside, though in a slightly less scary aspect of it.

I know what it feels like to be a parent who is worried stiff, who feels distrustful of the decisions that medical experts are making about her child, who would like to trust her instincts but never had anyone say that it's okay, in fact a good idea, to do just that.

So I'm going to start saying it to whoever will listen. In fact, I have already started. For the past few months I've been producing a newsletter for a microcephaly support group, which has 450 families in its membership.

There was a plea in the first newsletter I was sent soon after joining the group, for someone to take over as editor. I thought, "I can do that." But I hesitated. I was nervous of the commitment; I might regret it later. But then I rang anyway, and Annie, the coordinator, was grateful that I did.

It's been easy enough for me to do. But the project, to my surprise, has given me a real buzz. I love creating something that says whatever you feel is okay. It's great to offer positive encouragement.

And I enjoy talking to other members on the phone, having the odd meeting, reading the letters that come in. Sometimes I feel good because I'm helping other parents. Other times, they make me feel good, by giving me hope and encouragement. The letters are so full of strength and wisdom; I wish everyone in the world could read them.

I've also just signed a contract with Sheldon Press to write a 'how to' book, *Coping when Your Child has Special Needs*. It's a project that has more than a touch of serendipity about it.

The Sheldon Press book catalogue arrived one day in the post. I am on the mailing list because from time to time I write reviews of new publications.

I realised that many of the titles were about coping with various problems. And then I realised, to my surprise, that there wasn't a single book on the subject of special needs, or children's disabilities.

So I rang the press office. I spoke to a man who said they

didn't have anything like it in the pipeline, and the person to send a proposal to was the editorial director, Joanna Moriarty.

Her name made me blink because I knew her, a little. As new graduates, we had college friends in common. We occasionally met up, a group of us, in West End pubs. Then, years later, she was at Sheldon and I was at *New Woman* magazine, and I used to ring her for authors to interview, and for book extracts to publish in the magazine.

I'd heard that she'd become editorial director, but then I'd forgotten about it, until now. Jo was open to my book proposal, and it's fun working with her. We're both keen on the book that I'm writing. There is definitely a need for it.

"How do you have the energy for it?" asks my friend Julie at one of our group's weekly lunches. She's being kind. As always, I feel grateful for her support and that of the group.

The truth is, sometimes I don't have the energy. Some weeks I'm full of great ideas to share with other parents. Other times, like this minute right now, I wish that I could just be a willing disciple of a teacher who's active already in this field.

But the bottom line is this: each of us has our own life work to do. We may well overlap with others, but ultimately we each have our own individual tasks. So although there are many teachers and other parents who can give me help and inspiration, there is no one doing exactly what I've started to do.

When I look around, I see plenty of kind, energetic and impassioned people who are working to improve the rights of disabled people, and I totally go along with what they are doing.

But the 'how to' book that I'm writing is more of a practical encouragement for parents to use their intuition; and to believe in themselves and their children.

I am saying, "You and your child are normal, and your feelings are your best guide."

As I write this, at the end of the 20th century, it feels exactly as though I am standing in front of an unploughed field. The soil is very fertile. All I've got to do is start ploughing.

To be honest, it feels a bit embarrassing, starting the first furrows. Whatever will my friends think, when they read this book of dreams? We are not used, as a society, to revealing our inner worlds.

Then I remember Brian Duppa, who built a set of fine almshouses in Richmond because he remembered the vows he made to God in his trouble.

The really interesting thing is, other people followed his example. I don't know if you've ever been to Richmond, but it's full of almshouses. Several are laid around courtyards, like Cambridge colleges for senior citizens.

The first person to spend his money in this way might have felt a bit embarrassed. But then, it became quite the thing to do. A fashion for kindness was created that lasted two centuries and more, right up to the present day.

Although no one builds almshouses here anymore, I think the effects of kindness do accumulate in a community. Richmond is a kind and prospering place, unusually so for a London borough. People are likely to smile at you in the street if you catch their eye. Neighbours frequently say to each other, "It's so nice living here."

The primary schools came top in the national tables this year, and the borough has the highest number of graduates in the country. There is a feeling here of many people living fulfilling lives, and a liberal acceptance of differences.

When I think about it, I don't think we could have landed anywhere better to get us through our difficult times. True, our families mostly live some distance away, but they are great at moral support over the phone, and we do see them regularly. Beyond family, however, all the support we've needed has been here, and most of it within walking distance.

We've had wonderful helpers. One who really stands out is Elaine Gibson, our Portage home visitor. She comes once a week to help Timmy through play. She has listened to me patiently, many times, as I work out exactly what I think and feel about his challenges, and the wider world of cognitive and physical disabilities.

That role of listening is invaluable. How brilliant it would be if 'listening' were written into the job descriptions of all health professionals.

Other individuals such as Emma, our speech and language therapist, and Kerry, our occupational therapist, have come regularly and treated Timmy with real kindness. They've had some excellent ideas and insights, but have not been overly intrusive in the process.

Timmy's nursery, Monty's, has been a huge force for good. He goes there part-time while I do a certain amount of freelance writing. Tracy Mabbs, the owner, has been brilliant: kind, supportive, inclusive and capable.

Tracy has created a lovely welcoming space for young children. She and her staff, Phyllis, Irene, Alison, Rhiannydd and the others, have always been very keen to help Timmy in every way. We can tell that he loves being with them, and with the other children there. "A home from home," is how speech therapist Emma described it.

At the beginning of this year, a local charity called the Hampton Fuel Allotment Fund awarded Timmy a grant to pay for one-to-one help while he's at the nursery. So nowadays Linda Gregory comes in and is fantastic with him: together with gentle Rhiannydd, she helps him to do everything as independently as possible, so he feels like one of the group.

Timmy's very happy there, and he gets on well with the other children who are completely accepting of him. Especially since Linda's arrival, we've seen him grow in confidence and strength.

All this kindness and support, feeding into our situation… it does make a difference. And it feels natural to share and channel that strength towards others who are on their own path of personal development, whether that be through the lessons of cognitive disabilities, life-threatening illness, or perhaps some other wake-up call. I believe that many of us, perhaps all of us, have these wake-up calls, sooner or later.

The missing piece of jewellery

Long ago, in my early 20s, I dreamed I was walking along a dusty, warm country road, such as you might find in a sleepy part of Italy or, perhaps, in England during a long, hot summer.

I came to a beautiful large house, with wonderful gardens, well-tended yet natural. In the gardens there was a fountain, sparkling in the sunlight, and many young adults. They all seemed to be healthy, glowing and beautiful in the way that young people can be.

However, the young people were upset. They were searching for something. Several of them explained that the old lady, whose house this was, and whom they loved, had lost her piece of jewellery.

"What does it look like?" I asked, wanting to help.

"We're not sure what it was exactly, but she always wore it over her chest," one of the young people said. "It was gold."

And then I felt suddenly that I *could* help, because on my journey I had found some jewellery on the road and picked it up. So they took me inside to see the old lady. I didn't think she was old at all: she looked to be in her 60s or 70s. Or it may have been that she simply had a youthful air. She seemed serene, and not at all upset to have lost her jewellery. The room was decorated in gentle shades of gold, and her clothes were like that too. Altogether, it felt like a lovely place to be.

I went up to her and offered her the jewellery that I'd found on the way.

She looked at it, and smiled. All of a sudden I understood that this wasn't her jewellery at all. It was actually made of some base metal. It was not the real thing.

I felt abashed. Without saying a word to me, she'd just taught me a valuable lesson.

There was something else unsaid, but plainly evident: I felt that the older lady was an older version of myself. I was very happy with this realisation. I understood that my future self could act as a wise guide to me, and that she cared for me. It was a warm feeling. I woke up happy, though with a perplexing mystery: what exactly did the missing piece of jewellery signify?

When that dream occurred in my early 20s I had just split up from a boyfriend – actually, he had dumped me. I told him about the dream, and he said it was about the competitive element between the two of us.

It's true that we were competitive, which was one reason why we were never going to last as a couple. But I couldn't see that had anything to do with the dream.

Several years later, I met Steven. In the early weeks of knowing him, I told him the dream, because it was important to me and I was still trying to work out the meaning. Soon afterwards, for my 30th birthday, he gave me a gold necklace with a card that said, "The real thing."

It was a beautiful gift, and the love it represented seemed to tie in closely with the dream, but it still wasn't the whole answer.

And then, just recently, I was thinking about the dream again and suddenly I got it – a real 'aha' moment. The reason the old lady wasn't unhappy was because *she hadn't lost the gold jewellery at all*. It had simply become transformed. It was no longer a badge that she wore, but something that permeated her, and her surroundings. And Steven had been right: it was love.

The young people in the older lady's garden were learning about unconditional love and self-acceptance simply by being in the older lady's presence. They were glowing in her light, and in their own inner light.

My future self wasn't giving the young people advice. She was simply being herself. In the process, she was creating a peaceful space for other people to be themselves. In their turn they were becoming a light to others.

My future self somehow taught me this: the kindest thing we can do for others is simply be ourselves. It's what we're best at.

We all have special needs. We're all vulnerable. We all deserve oodles of extra loving care. And we all need to give that to ourselves as well as to others.

Here is my wish: to help people to move through their challenges and reconnect with themselves: to know that they are normal and perfect, just as they are.

Here is how I do it: through writing. Writing can be therapeutic, empowering and healing.

Sometimes I think I would like us to live in a peaceful old house, as the older lady of my dream did, where others could come and relax and be themselves. There'd be a lovely scented garden to enjoy, and a library full of good books. They'd be able to talk to like-minded souls and share experiences.

It would be a place for people to do what they want to do, not what others tell them to do. To encourage this outlook there might even be a plaque by the front door, saying something that Steven once wrote on a gold-coloured gift tag, tied to his very first present to me: *"Dum vivimus vivamus,"* which means, 'While we live, let us live'.

I still have that gift tag: it's here on the desk as I write. The actual present – a box of chocolates – vanished just as quickly as chocolates should.

Maybe the house would be in Richmond, where people could go to the cinema or theatre. They'd be able to walk in the magical oak woodlands and bracken meadows of Richmond Park, watching the deer graze. Or they'd visit the botanical riches of Kew Gardens, and tune into the wisdom of the plants there. And they'd walk along the silvery Thames, maybe even take a boat trip....

Or perhaps the house would be in the English countryside,

along a beautiful rustic track. People visiting would feel that they were leaving their cares and duties behind. They would have a chance simply to be themselves in the company of like-minded souls.

Who knows what, if any, of this will happen? But having a vision, and keeping it, and taking it out and looking at it from time to time, like a treasured photo, is the best way I know of reaching the right future for me.

14. Three gifts

So what have I learned from all of this? Perhaps most of it comes down to three simple insights, which I have tucked into my toolbox of strategies.

1. Respect your feelings

The first insight is to respect my feelings. I need to listen to my intuition. There is a pattern to my life, but I can't see it, except in occasional glimpses, if I am lucky. My intuition will help me to progress even when I can't logically see the way.

It's as if I am walking over my own beautiful, woven rug. The rug is so vast, it would take a lifetime to cover it all. It takes such a long time partly because I do not walk consistently in a straight line, from one end to the next. Sometimes I stop still. Other times, I go sideways or even backwards.

Now here is the magical thing. The woven rug is blank until I walk upon it. Wherever my footsteps go, pattern is created.

The pattern is a reflection of my feelings and actions.

Perhaps I go through a sad time. It feels then as though I am walking in circles. Although I don't realise it, the pattern that is left might be a beautiful, subtle bluish-grey, with lots of overlapping circles that look like petals from above.

A few months later, I am full of joy and dancing. The pattern that my footsteps leave is a light, joyous one of golden flower shapes.

When I fall out with someone, angular black lines might be created. When I experience love, a rose pink colour suffuses the area in which I walk.

I cannot see the effect of my actions and feelings. To do so, I'd have to fly high above the rug, like a bird – or a soul on its way back to heaven. However, if I could see my rug in its entirety, I would know that there are no mistakes. Whatever the pattern of my rug, it is beautiful. It is the pattern of me doing my very best to learn about life. Ultimately, it is a pattern of love.

To realise the true tapestry of my life while I am still walking its path, my feelings are my best guide. They will take me to places where logic would never dream of going. I can be sure of this, because logic never dreams.

But I *can* dream, and my dreams will point me in the right direction for me, which is never exactly the same as anyone else's direction. We all live according to our own pattern – a pattern that we create.

The more I listen to my dreams, the more I discover that they often point to my future, and the futures of those I love. In this sense, dreams can transport me above the beautiful woven rug of my life. In my dreams every night and sometimes during the day, I can fly high above the pattern. I can get a longer perspective; see two weeks, two years or even more into the future.

Often my feelings tell me things that don't seem to fit in with the overall pattern of my life. I need to trust these feelings. The pattern is never a grid, with straight lines leading forwards and sideways. I am not totally in control, even though I sometimes like to think I am. There are unexpected curves. In time, I see these were essential for the overall shape of the design.

Some of the curves involve intuitive decisions that seem crazy at the time, but they make perfect sense in the long run.

Here is one example. Ten years ago, in 1989, I was an associate editor on *New Woman* magazine. It was a good job. However, I really wanted to be a freelance writer, but didn't dare make the leap, because I didn't have any savings to support me while I built up my new income.

Suddenly, from nowhere, I was overcome by a strong urge to work on a tabloid newspaper. I simply had to do it. It was obvious to me that I was not the right material for that kind of job. But even so, I had to do it.

I went to see three tabloid editors. My own magazine editor

immediately heard about this through the journalistic grapevine. She told me that she was planning to move to a tabloid herself, to edit its Sunday magazine. There was room for me if I'd like to come along. So I did.

The editorial offices on Fleet Street were shabby and grandiose in equal measure. It felt like a tired old empire whose days were numbered. Insecurity was rife. I felt very uncomfortable there, but still felt that I was 'on track' in ways I couldn't understand. However, I was pretty sure that I wasn't going to be there for long. I used to look at some of the older journalists and see how lined with stress their faces had become. Frankly, I didn't want to stick around and start looking similarly stressed.

My editor had a plan to bring the magazine upmarket through a management buyout. The buyout was chancy. Before I was hired, she told me that if it didn't work, I could either accept another job at the newspaper company, presuming one was available; or take six months' pay as part of a tax-free redundancy package.

The buyout didn't happen. Six months after I arrived, the day it all fell through, the editor was telling me to ring this person or that in the group, to make sure I got a decent replacement job. I picked up the phone obediently.

But then, a quiet, firm voice in me said, "Put down that phone!"

And so I did. I went into the editor's office and said, "Actually, I'd rather take the redundancy package."

I found it hard to say those words. I was *so* used to sticking with the flock. In those days I scarcely ever thought of speaking my truth. I lacked confidence. But once I'd said my bit, the rest was easy. I had made the leap, and suddenly, I had become my own person.

My salary in the newspaper group was higher than I'd been used to, so the redundancy package felt satisfyingly large.

After I'd left the paper, I looked back at the whole experience in some amazement. Yes, I'd gained some interesting experience. I'd learned more about myself. If nothing else, I knew what I didn't want to do.

But I'd got the cash cushion that I'd been looking for.

I wondered if, on a subliminal level, my brief sojourn at a tabloid empire had been mainly about that.

A more recent example of listening to my feelings came about when Steven and I suddenly decided to take Timmy to the Caribbean. During the weeks before we went, before we even knew we were going, I had a whole series of dreams suggesting that travel was imminent.

In my waking hours, I was overcome by a strong urge to travel: I simply had to travel, even though for the past three years I had been happy to stay in Richmond with occasional trips to the country.

Steven was ready for us to go. It's fair to say that Steven is always ready to travel. And so we made the leap, we took our vulnerable son to the Caribbean, and the warm sunshine helped him in ways that were wonderful to see. It felt like a watershed, a turning point for him.

2. Do what you want to do

The second lesson I've learned is to be led by pleasure, not duty. Pleasure comes from doing the thing that is right for me, whatever that may be. Duty is doing what other people think I should do.

Other people are often wrong.

We are taught much more about what we should or shouldn't do, than about the importance of enjoying ourselves. Why have we got it so topsy-turvy? Pleasure is not selfish, or harmful to others. Pleasure very often involves caring for others. I can get huge enjoyment from going shopping and finding an appropriate gift for someone. But if I view the task as a duty, the pleasure is stripped away and the present becomes a grudging one.

When I deprive myself of pleasure on a daily basis, I develop cravings. "I shan't eat chocolate," I say, "because I shouldn't. It's bad for me." And so I think about the chocolate longingly, and sooner or later I have a splurge, and then I feel guilty, and I vow to deprive myself even more. But the more I deprive myself, the more liable I am to splurge, sooner or later.

The body is its own self-regulator. Left to its own devices, the body will eat lots of chocolate at first because it's reacting against the previous restrictions. But then it will simply go off it. We can trust our appetite, as long as we are not distorting it by squashing our natural feelings.

When Timmy was born, duty told Steven and me that we should take our son to endless medical appointments that seldom seemed to do any good. Duty told us that we should force him to endure endless painful tests involving needles, anaesthetics and worse... Duty insisted this was the right thing to do, even though the tests never led to a practical solution but caused a lot of grief and even damage in the process. In consequence, Timmy has developed a phobia about all medical situations – even the helpful ones.

Duty told us that we should follow the therapist's advice when she said we should put our son in a standing frame, even though we could see that he became quiet and withdrawn. Duty also said we should give him antibiotics every day, just to be on the safe side, even though they gave him diarrhoea and rashes, and killed the beneficial flora in his intestines.

Pleasure says, "No," to all these things. Pleasure says, "Stuff duty, let's be happy! Let's go on holiday and cancel the medical appointments that happen to fall in that fortnight! Forget therapy exercises today, let's go swimming instead!"

Pleasure says, "Live life to the full."

Duty says, "Live life according to other people's rules."

Which would you rather do? I want to shout it from the

rooftops: "IT'S MY CHOICE!"

3. Remember that we are all connected

The third lesson I've learned is that we are all connected. Recently I came across a personal diary that I kept when I was a staff journalist. My life then was a round of social gatherings in wine bars, careerist ambition and, at regular intervals to escape it all, travel.

I'm shocked at how spiritually empty and isolated it all seems now. Looking back, I see how brittle I was then, how much I kept myself separate from others. I loved my family and friends, but everyone else was outside the bubble. Actually, on some basic level, even my family and friends were outside the bubble. I was the only one in it.

I remember that time when we travelled north to Oldham, to Steven's warm-hearted family for Christmas shortly after he and I first met. As we left the motorway in the dusk and the snow, I began to look at the houses we passed with a new awareness. They seemed more decorated than their southern counterparts. Many had flashing lights in the windows, and I saw countless Christmas trees visible through draped net curtains.

It struck me then: each of those homes belonged to little circles of love and friendship, and there were countless such circles, not just on our route, but across the globe.

It was a moment of awareness that paved the way for a more open-hearted attitude within me.

Becoming a parent can have this effect anyway, I suspect. Becoming a parent of a child with health issues multiplies the potential for worry and fear – for suffering. And suffering in one sphere of life can be just what is required to open the heart. Once the heart is open, it's easy to feel empathy for all people who suffer, in myriad ways.

Everyone experiences deep sadness, sooner or later. This might manifest as bereavement, or abandonment, or feeling alone, or dealing with a loved one's illness, or drifting apart from someone we once loved… there are many variations available. There are also countless smaller disappointments along the way.

In the way I deal with my sources of grief, I have a choice. I can either learn the lesson of empathy and connection, or I can close up and say, "This is not happening."

It's possible to spot the people who choose the path of denial. They close up emotionally. They develop a tight-lipped, colourless look, with perhaps a brittle laugh. They don't talk their problems through. They might ask a barrage of questions rather than allow an opening into their own innermost feelings. That was me, as a journalist, all through my 20s and early 30s.

It's also possible to spot the people who learn the path of empathy. They are more open, relaxed… they're happier. They don't look short of love and hugs. They have a glow about them.

Deep down, they are kind to themselves. They have a sense of love and self-acceptance. That is hopefully me now, aged 38 – the mother of a young disabled child.

When I don't see the connection between myself and other people, there can be a tendency to demonise the others. The 'others' could be a group of people who happen to think differently to me. It could be a friend I have fallen out with, or a member of my own family. It could be a person who appears to have authority over me: a boss, a doctor, or a politician.

But I can be sure that the people I find challenging do not think of themselves in that way. In their world, I might well be the baddy, while they are the misunderstood heroes. When, in my magazine days, a particularly difficult boss used to snap at me, she undoubtedly believed she was in the right. She may genuinely have felt that I was a fool. Conversely, she might have feared that the ambitious younger woman who worked for her was after her job. So she felt insecure, and I felt insecure.

The answer is for me to look at 'difficult' people differently. Instead of thinking mean thoughts about a tactless medic, I might send a blessing. I can make a point of remembering that we are all connected. We are all at different points in a very complex, far-reaching and quite amazing whole. The medic is my sibling, parent, child, or cousin, and I am theirs.

This is a hard lesson to learn. I have found myself drifting between believing this, and not believing it. Over time, I believe it more and more. One day it may be second nature to me.

Once I started thinking in these terms, that we are all connected, I began to realise why disabled people shouldn't be segregated. Even anti-discrimination laws don't go far enough. It's not just about money and jobs. It's important that our hearts are also engaged. The disabled people I have met and known, every single one of them, are my brothers, sisters, parents and children. The same applies to any group of people, without exception. We are all kin.

Ultimately, when I help others, in a radical and deep-rooted way, I am holding out a hand to myself. I love and accept who I am. I don't have to be flawless. But I do truly need to be myself, and thus accept myself whole-heartedly.

Book Two

The Miracle Child Grows Up

Glimpses of Timothy up to eighteen years of age:
choosing confidence and freedom.

15. Moving to Wiltshire

Wiltshire, 2013. It's dawn. I have woken up with words for this chapter in my mind. They are jostling to be written down.

Steven and the children are all asleep. I pad down to the kitchen, top up the kettle with water, and place it back on the Aga. Bovril, our elderly black cat, comes to say, "Hello."

Bovril hasn't always lived with us. When we moved to this beautiful, breezy hill in Wiltshire, 11 years ago, we had no pets.

Soon after we moved in, we noticed a black cat would walk swiftly through our garden once a day, every day. After a few weeks of this, we noticed that he was walking more slowly. He began to stop and groom himself, then continue on his way.

After a while, the mysterious cat spent more and more time in our garden. He began to come up to us, and even follow us around. We discovered that he belonged to our neighbours, higher up on the hill. We learnt his name: Bovril. We started talking to him, and stroking him, but we didn't let him into the house and we didn't feed him.

Over the next few years, Bovril began to come into the house, but we still didn't feed him. Then one day Andrea, the wonderful lady who helps out with Tim and indeed the whole household, brought in a box of cat biscuits that her cat had rejected. "Bovril might as well have them," she said. And when that packet was finished, we bought another....

So, year by year, Bovril became more and more our cat. For the longest time, I felt ambivalent about this. He wasn't ours, and I didn't like the idea of taking him away from our neighbours, but he didn't seem to want to go back home, even though he was much loved there. The problem was that he didn't get on with that household's dogs.

I was also uncomfortably aware that a black cat could be viewed as a rather witchy thing. This hit a nerve, as some of my activities were also looking the teeniest bit pagan. I'm not the sort to cast spells. However, I was getting more and more into healing, intuitive development, and herb growing.

While we were still living in Richmond, around the time that I was completing the earlier part of this book, I studied spiritual healing at Richmond College with the NFSH Healing Trust, under the inspiring tutorship of Darryl O'Keeffe. The healing I learned and practised that year felt completely natural, as though I was connecting with 'the real me'. My sensitivity to people's emotions and energies, the remarkable intuitive insights I frequently received... these things were, I discovered, a normal part of spiritual healing, or energy healing as it is sometimes called. I was thrilled to be with like-minded people. It truly felt as though I had 'come home'.

On Wednesday evenings I used to join a team of volunteer healers at Richmond Healing Centre, run by a kindly married couple, Brian and May Franklin, where we gave healing to members of the public. The atmosphere there was peaceful and uplifting. I loved working with individuals and seeing how relaxed they were after a session. I remember the way one man with schizophrenia found his tormenting voices fell progressively silent over a series of sessions, and how he connected again with his estranged family. I remember one woman who had been unable to conceive, but did so after several healing sessions. I remember several fragile individuals with cancer who seemed to get such solace from the healing.

During part of that wonderful year of learning, I also studied herbal medicine at Richmond College, taught by herbalist Nina Nissen. I loved Nina's intelligence, passion for the subject, and lack of ego. Both Darryl and Nina had a profound influence on me, as did the kindly healers at Richmond Healing Centre. Metaphorically, full of gratitude, I lay fragrant roses at their doors.

After further training in Bath, Chippenham and Glastonbury,

I finally passed Panel in Blandford Forum and became accredited as a spiritual healer in 2003. Then people started coming to see me, either on a one-to-one basis for healing, or in small groups to meditate. The room we use has spectacular views over North Wiltshire, and a remarkably peaceful atmosphere. Surrounded by nature, it's perfect for the purpose.

The herbal medicine was mainly on a friends and family basis, although I also started making rainwater soaps and balms with herbs from the hedgerows. While our daughter was young, I used to sell these at local fundraisers under the name of Dream Botanicals.

So, with the herbs and the healing combined, I felt that in some ways it could be thought that I was entering witch territory, and it seemed that a black cat was just rubbing this in. I didn't want to be witchlike. Then one day I looked up the origins of the word, and discovered that 'witch' originally meant 'wise woman, one who sees'. That made the presence of a black cat seem a little better, but I still felt ambivalent.

But time is a wonderful thing. Quite simply, we all got used to each other. Even Steven, who is not so fond of animals, was heard calling Bovril "darling" one day.

A few years ago, our neighbours officially handed Bovril over to us, which changed things. It felt easy to bond with him then. Nowadays, at the age of 17, Bovril spends much of his time by the warm Aga in the kitchen. He's a constant little companion and we are all very fond of him. He has become a special presence in our family. Our daughter Grace, who is eight years younger than Tim, adores him. It's mainly her job to feed him.

So, it's early morning in the kitchen, and I am making myself a cup of herbal tea: marshmallow leaf with lemon verbena. It's just a few days since I rediscovered and read the manuscript for *The Miracle Child*. I am still mulling over the contents.

The verbena fills the air with a beautiful citrus fragrance. Through the wisps of steam, I feel as though the younger me is just behind me, urging me on. She is saying, "Only believe."

But only believe in what, exactly? The answer comes instantly. This isn't about religious beliefs. It's simpler than that.

I must believe in Tim, and in his innate healing ability. That same ability runs through all living beings, and through all the atoms of the universe. It's a force for life: a powerful current, electrifying and animating all matter that it touches.

Only believe. Belief opens the doors and lets the current flow.

Acute senses

As Tim has grown, he has changed. He has become more grounded, more fully in his body. Some of his more other-worldly characteristics have diminished. These used to be considerable. For example, when Tim was little he used to spend a lot of time in La-la Land, as we called it. He chatted, laughed, and gazed at things invisible to us, often at a level slightly above him. It's rare for him to do that during the daytime now – though he still does it, especially late at night, when he sometimes appears to be having a bit of a party while lying in bed.

Tim also used to exhibit some interesting and unusual abilities. As I mentioned earlier, when he was three, his nursery moved location and we suddenly had quite a long walk to reach it. Sometimes I cycled, but most of the time I walked, pushing Tim in the buggy in front of me. Our journey took us across a railway line. It was a busy line, with lots of trains going through. Often, the gates would be closed, and we would have to wait for a train. To pass the time I would play a little game with him. I expect parents the world over play a similar game.

"Can you guess which direction the train will come from, Timmy?" I would ask him.

He would point, to the right or to the left. *And he was right every single time.* This went on for many months. If this was coincidence, it was an astonishing one. It seemed for all the world as though Tim's senses could tell unerringly from which direction the train was coming, even when the train was still a long way away.

His apparent hypersensitivity concerning trains began to diminish around a year later. Shortly before he left Monty's, just before he started school, he started to get it wrong sometimes. Concurrently, he was becoming a little more settled in his body, a little more grounded.

There was another version of this game, however, that lasted far longer. We used to put a small object such as a pebble in one hand, then hold both closed hands out in front of him. "Which hand is it in, Tim?" we would ask. And for years on end, into his early teens, he chose correctly each time. But gradually that too started to vanish. As it did, he appeared more and more grounded in his own body. Now, it has completely gone.

There is, however, one heightened sensitivity that Tim still exhibits. Sometimes I will think something, and he will answer it before I've even spoken the words. For example, I might think: "Perhaps we could go for a drive today." And Tim will sign, "Yes, please." And then he will say "Car," and he will sign it too, all with a big, expectant smile. (Tim loves car journeys.)

He will do all of this even though I have not spoken a single word.

Tim also remains hyper-aware of people's emotions, and new things that enter the house. He is simply *aware*. In the old days, he would take things in with peripheral vision. He avoided eye contact. Nowadays he still uses peripheral vision more than most people might. However, often he is simply still, watching directly with bright eyes.

What I have just written about hypersensitivity would be laughed out of any medical room. Or, at best, it would be politely ignored. But Tim is not the only young person with disabilities to show unusual sensory behaviour. I've been privileged to meet many such people over the years, each with their own unique sensory neural configuration. It's such a shame that this area is not more fully studied, and acknowledged.

Only believe.

Tim has thrived when I have believed in him. This is how it works: when I believe in him, he believes in himself. The whole family believes in him. There is more laughter in the house.

When I don't believe in him, there is less laughter. When I don't believe in him, the doomsayers' predictions appear to be true. He does not thrive.

And then I believe again, and he thrives again. His colour returns, and the fun returns.

Only believe.

Wherever you are, whatever you are dealing with, please do this: *believe.* Believe in yourself; believe in your loved ones. Believe that life is fun and you all can thrive.

No regrets

As the herbal tea gently brews, there is a question in my mind that I need to answer.

What would I do differently? If I could visit my younger self, what would I say to her?

The answers come rushing.

Above all, I would trust myself. I would value my intuition. I would consider it a divine tool to help me navigate a happier path.

I would be kinder to myself. I would listen to my body and respond to the signals of exhaustion and stress. I would allow myself to rest. I would value my own ability to make good decisions for my own well-being, and that of Tim.

I would develop my own unique toolkit of strategies to help me when I felt low.

The herbal tea is ready now. Outside, the sky is turning silvery grey. A wood pigeon is cooing somewhere nearby. I take a few sips of the tea and feel its gentle warmth spread throughout my body. The marshmallow leaf, from our garden, creates a subtle, smooth, full texture. The lemon verbena, from my parents' greenhouse, is fragrant and uplifting.

The truth is I did develop that toolkit. I wrote a book, *Coping when Your Child has Special Needs*. It sold a modest number of copies. I got some lovely letters from other parents who said it was their bible.

And of course I trained as a healer. And along the way I developed a way of meditating intuitively that I now enjoy sharing with others.

Would I have done those things if Tim had been born without major health issues?

As I type those words, the familiar sadness returns. The sorrow is clearly still a part of my life. How lovely it would have been if Tim had been born healthy, and grown up healthy.

My original group of post-natal friends has dispersed now, but we stay in touch in a gentle, low-key way, still supportive, mainly online. Every now and then I see photos of their children. Some of the images show them outdoors, hiking. Last year there was a scattering of prom photos. When I see such a photo, there is always a slight pang. I feel happiness for the teenager pictured, and their family. I feel sadness for mine.

And then I remind myself that we are so lucky Tim is still here.

Over many years of intermittent chest infections, Tim's spinal curvature has become more complex. It is now his biggest challenge. It's harder and harder for him to breathe deeply enough, and for the past year, since the age of 16, he has started having supplementary oxygen at night and through some of the day, delivered from a portable cylinder via a small respiratory mask.

I think back to that brace fitting at Great Ormond Street Hospital. If we could make the decision again, would we have made him wear a brace? After all, he was very young. He needn't have had any say in it.

I'm typing this at a table in the hall. It's small and oak-lined, one of my favourite rooms in this peaceful home of ours.

On the wall opposite, there is a remarkable painting that was created by our talented friend, the lettering artist Caroline Keevil. I gave it as a birthday present to Steven a few years back. It has special meaning for the whole family. In golden letters against a swirly red and gold background are the words: *Dum Vivimus Vivamus* – the words Steven originally wrote for me on that gift tag over 20 years ago. The painted gold is real.

While we live, let us live.

At the time of the brace fitting, we knew a little girl of Tim's age who had similar problems with her spine. Her mother once said to me that her daughter had the same issues Tim had, but a little bit worse. The little girl was quieter than Tim. She moved her body as if in slow motion, compared with his quicksilver movements. She was sweet and lovely to be with. Somehow, like Tim, she still seemed to have that open connection with heaven.

That little girl did wear a back brace. And that little girl died very early on, from pneumonia.

Steven and I have always believed that Tim, like us, should live life to the full. His present-day community paediatrician, a wise and gentle lady, said to me recently that we have never 'medicalised' Tim. She clearly meant it as a compliment.

Tim has a varied and stimulating life. He loves travel of any sort.

Just like his dad, in fact.

Steven did follow up his interest in flying, after the Everest trip he went on in the late 90s. Today, he flies planes and helicopters, to help others and for amazing adventures.

A few weeks ago, for example, he flew from England to America via Iceland, Greenland and Canada in a small, single-engined plane.

He is also a pilot trustee for a charity called fly2help that gives young people with health and other issues a chance to experience the freedom of flying.

As a family, we have also had huge, adventurous fun in the sky. We have soared in a small plane over the mountains of Norway to Bergen. We have flown over the Alps to Salzburg. We have swooped low over the Venetian Lagoon, and skirted the glittering blue bay of Cannes.

And Tim has loved it all. He still gets really excited about it. As talking is largely beyond him, he uses signs. And the sign for 'plane' is one of his favourites.

Tim enjoys gazing out at the earth receding beneath him as we take off. He enjoys the 'white noise' and vibration of the engine while we fly. He sometimes sings to himself as he looks out into space, at the vast blue expanse above the clouds. He usually holds his favourite 'taggie' on his lap, a soft toy shaped like a rugby ball, with silken loops that his fingers constantly touch. And he looks with interest at the earth, rushing to meet him as we land.

Would we do anything differently? Would we put our two-year-old son in a back brace 23 hours a day? Would we give him an MRI scan? Would we strap him into a walking frame?

No, no and no. The truth is, we wouldn't, because we did the best we knew how at the time.

Medical approaches vary from one year to the next. Medical beliefs are presented as an absolute truth, but then the belief changes to another absolute truth.

Tim has taught me to listen to my intuition.

Every child is a teacher to the parent.

By the time Tim's baby sister came along, my parenting style had become more natural and confident. I breastfed Tim for 19 months, and I'm so glad I did. But I breastfed Grace for double that time, and I'm equally glad about that. I carried Tim some of the time in a baby carrier. I carried Grace routinely in a sling, and scarcely used a buggy. Tim slept in our bed quite often, when he was poorly or just in need of hugs. Grace was born in our bed and had no other bed until she was 19 months old.

When Tim was a baby, I was very distrustful of medical professionals, whom I saw as flawed and arrogant leaders of a discredited health system. Today, I realise that on a deeper level they were mirrors to my own inner turmoil. Today I have less turmoil, and I get on reasonably well with most of Tim's varied health professionals. I value them more fully, from the heart. But I never make the mistake of thinking they have the final answer. I think their vision is blinkered.

I still get frustrated by a system that I perceive wants us to exaggerate Tim's disabilities in order to get the financial help to do this or that.

However, even on my worst days I know that sending unconditional love and blessing into any situation transforms it. It really does. It has become second nature to do this, and I share that exercise with many of the people who come to me for healing.

Above all, I have learned that we need to love and accept ourselves. Doing this creates a deep, still, calm peace inside us. This peace is deeply transformative. When I feel that peace, my own inner wisdom returns to me. This wisdom, or intuition, is my compass. I see it as the voice of the greater part of me that is plugged into the Divine. The intuitive part of me is not separate. It doesn't live solely in my physical frame. It is part of an infinite whole.

The voice within certainly helps me through tricky bits along my life path. But I can only hear that voice when I'm in a loving space. So I make a point of meditating regularly to keep and cultivate that sense of calm within me.

Until I learnt to access my own inner peace, I could never begin to trust other people. I saw them as 'other'. Without my own inner wisdom, I was looking to others for answers. But they were not living my life. Therefore, however many exams they had passed, they could never navigate my course as well as I could.

Most importantly of all, I have learned – am still learning – to trust in the power of love, the guidance of the Divine, and the interconnectedness of all beings.

Three texts from very different sources reached me today that neatly reflect the above words that I wrote this morning.

The first was a comment by Emmet Fox, a spiritual writer from the 20th century. This is how it goes:

There is no difficulty that enough love will not conquer. There is no disease that enough love will not heal. No door that enough love will not open. No gulf that enough love will not bridge. No wall that enough love will not throw down. And no sin that enough love will not redeem. It makes no difference how deeply seated may be the trouble. How hopeless the outlook. How muddled the tangle. How great the mistake. A sufficient realization of love will dissolve it all. And if you could love enough you would be the happiest and most powerful person in the world.

The message there is clear: whatever question or difficulty you may have, love is the answer.

The second text I read today was a comment on Eternea, the website devoted to spiritually transformative experiences (STEs) co-founded by Dr Eben Alexander, who underwent a near-death experience and wrote it up in his book, *Proof of Heaven*:

STEs often create difficult challenges for the experiencer until the experience can be completely integrated into one's life.

That resonates with me. I had a blissful mystical vision, followed by a most challenging experience of parenting a child with complex disabilities. I have learned so much already… and I continue to learn, every day of my life.

The third text I read came home in Grace's school bag this afternoon. She had been given a story to read that she considered laughably simple. "Just look at it, Mummy," she said. "Look how big the writing is!"

I read the title: *Mrs Maginty and the Cornish Cat* by Ann Jungman. I opened the book. My daughter was right: the writing was huge compared with the novels she reads at home. But the story was a pleasing one of magic and healing. And this is what I read:

Once people are touched by the magic and see things and themselves in a different way, they never return to their old ways.

When I was studying spiritual healing, in Richmond, one of my sponsors suggested I go to see a psychic. I had never consulted one before. Even picking up the phone to make the appointment at the College of Psychic Studies seemed 'woo woo'.

On the day, I managed to turn up late. Part of me simply didn't want to be there. However, I liked the atmosphere in the College, and its location in South Kensington. I was drawn to the library on the ground floor, which appeared to be full of fascinating books. I would have liked to study them. Instead, I was sent immediately upstairs to a small consulting room.

The psychic, Dr Angela Martin, got my attention straight away. She said that someone close to me had died a short while before, of a brain haemorrhage. This was totally accurate: so sadly, my older sister had died in just that way a few months earlier. We were very close, and missing her was a sharp, physical pain.

I asked Angela about my son and she had difficulty tuning into him at first. She asked me to talk about his medical condition. I didn't want to, but I listed the words anyway: microcephaly, scoliosis, global delays, and hypotonia... The energy in the room seemed to move downwards with the medical language.

Angela was able to 'tune in' to him on that level. But she explained that he seemed far away.

"There will be no miracles," said Angela. "He is the miracle." She added that she saw him doing lots of physiotherapy, and it would help him.

Of course, I didn't like that one bit. I wanted to hear that he would get better. I wanted to be told that he would lose all his difficulties and become indistinguishable from every other 'normal' person on the planet.

I was also falling into the trap – again – of believing that someone else held the answers.

The truth is, we *have* seen endless miracles along the way. There have been some big ones, and many little ones. In Chapter One I mentioned the time in Richmond when there was a potentially dangerous accident. A metal-framed camp bed fell down heavily on top of Tim's thin legs. He made a little noise of surprise. That was all.

Hardly daring to breathe, I lifted the camp bed from his legs. Although the metal frame had come down hard and fast, there was not a single mark on his legs.

Another time, years later in Wiltshire (I don't like thinking about this), I accidentally left the brakes off his wheelchair.

Tim's chair wheeled down the yard – with him in it – and toppled over. We ran after him and lifted him carefully. There was, again, no mark.

In an essential way, however, Angela was right: *Tim is the miracle*. He is a light in our lives. He has created happiness, harmony and plenty of laughter all around him. Our family is so much happier for having him in it. My heart has opened. By that, I mean that I can connect with others empathetically and feel compassion in a way I wasn't able to before. I thought I did. But it was nothing compared with what I can feel today.

There are also, increasingly, signs that physio could be very helpful for him. His legs, although thin, are strong in their way.

However, at the time of writing, we have not yet found a way of enabling him to have good, consistent exercise.

The world is what you make it

When Tim was six years old, just before we moved to Wiltshire, I had a short yet curious dream. In the dream, Steven and I were standing on either side of a large globe of the world. It was on a table between us. We were shaping the globe with our hands and it was continuously changing shape under our hands. It stayed spherical, but it was elastic and malleable.

There was a happy feeling in the dream – real joy. The message was clear to me: the world is what you make it. Nothing is set in stone, contrary to what we may think. Our thoughts and actions shape the world as surely as a ceramist can shape a lump of clay.

The message of the dream was overwhelmingly positive. It was celebrating something that Steven and I were just discovering in real life: happy thoughts create a happy world.

Focus on qualities such as fun, love, laughter, community, compassion and companionship. And the world you create will contain bundles of those same components.

And then we found an old stone house in the countryside. It was the sort of place I dreamed of living in when I was a child. The house seemed like a sanctuary: a place to put down roots.

Going to school in the Wild West

Starting Tim at the local village school was... interesting. Previously, Tim had been at a mainstream school, The Vineyard in Richmond, with one-to-one support. There were challenges, but overall it worked well.

The most important thing about Richmond was that he felt happy and included. The Vineyard is popular with expat families. Many nationalities were represented. True, Tim's disabilities made him noticeably different, but being German, Italian or Greek made other classmates somewhat different too.

There was a delightful culture in Richmond of differences being completely normal. People were friendly, gregarious and accepting. The diversity of people created lots of buzzy, interesting conversations. Socially there were lots of children's parties and play dates, and Tim was included in many of those. It was a happy time.

We had a Statement of Special Educational Needs, which spelled out that Tim was entitled to one-to-one support in a mainstream setting. This was a valuable legal document.

Getting the Statement in Richmond had been relatively straightforward. I remember before Tim started at school, an educational psychologist assessed him. She visited him in his nursery. She was very struck by how the other children loved playing with him, and how Tim smiled and responded to them. She said he should attend mainstream school because he was so sociable. He was therefore likely to benefit from a mainstream setting – as long as he had the right support.

In Richmond there was a peripatetic team of special needs teaching assistants. They did brilliant work helping children like Tim access mainstream schooling. They were professionals in their own right. They benefited from regular training sessions together, led by their very able manager. During those sessions they would pool their experiences and hone their skills.

In contrast, Wiltshire had nothing like that. Schools hired their own special needs TAs when required. But there weren't that many such TAs. At that time in Wiltshire, children with complex physical and learning disabilities always went to special schools.

Tim's Statement from liberal Richmond, a legal, binding document, meant that he was entitled to be educated in a mainstream school with one-to-one support.

When we decided to move, we applied to the local village school in Wiltshire, and they accepted him. They were open and willing to learn what they could do to help this unusual new pupil who couldn't walk and couldn't even talk, apart from a few sporadic words.

Before he left The Vineyard, the Special Educational Needs Coordinator from the village school made the 100-mile journey to visit him at The Vineyard, together with a TA. We were impressed and grateful that they made the journey.

It was shortly before Christmas. The usual timetable at The Vineyard had been dropped in favour of festivities. I'm not sure how much the two ladies learned in the circumstances. I just remember the faster children whizzing around as Tim looked on, entertained. But we were very grateful that they made the effort.

Despite their best efforts, Tim found the move to Wiltshire very hard. He cried when we left the house in Richmond for the last time. He looked around the empty living room with such sadness. He was almost seven. He couldn't talk beyond a few occasional words, but he could certainly understand.

Stepping into the village school in Wiltshire felt like stepping into a Wild West saloon bar. We were noticed. It seemed that everyone immediately knew who we were. Word had spread.

There were little reminders that we were different. A newsletter sent out to parents at that time warmly welcomed the arrival of a new teaching assistant, or TA, to look after an unnamed 'wheelchair-bound boy'. I was quietly outraged. There was no sense that he had an identity. There was no hint that he was also welcome.

We also, for the record, never considered that Tim was 'bound' to his wheelchair. He regularly took steps, with support. He could sit on normal chairs, or on the carpet.

When Tim first arrived at the school in January, the heating had failed, but no one mentioned that. The place was freezing, and I supposed that must be normal. Tim had to wear his coat indoors, he was so cold.

At lunchtimes, I had to collect Tim and bring him home for lunch every day, because the headmaster decided that the school could not cater for Tim's need for soft or puréed food.

After a couple of weeks, the school decided to put Tim in a younger class – actually two years below his chronological age. This was not an idea that had ever been broached in Richmond. I think it was fully understood in Richmond that Tim was never going to be able to keep up academically. How could he? The main benefit to him was social, and he got on very well with his peers.

However, we could see the village school's point of view, and we agreed to the move.

Subliminally, I could see that we baffled the headmaster, who was in his last year before retirement. For the whole of his own school career, disabled children had been segregated in special schools. In contrast, we were like exotic foreigners who didn't understand this age-old rule. But he was a kind man, and in his way he welcomed Tim.

The headmaster's big ambition for Tim was that he should learn the Lord's Prayer in sign language. It was, after all, a church school. Diligently, we practised the moves. But they didn't stick. It felt as though we were teaching Tim a trick. The long sequence was too abstract for Tim. After a while, the subject was quietly dropped.

Tim enjoyed learning signs, but preferred ones that represented things you could see or do. So he was quick to learn signs for animals – a favourite subject – as well as transport and food. The basics like 'yes', 'home', 'more', 'please', 'thank you' and 'tired' also featured frequently. He could also say a small number of words. What he said most often, many times a day, was, "Ready, steady, go!" This was fun, but didn't always go down too well with teachers during school assemblies.

There was a lot of kindness in the village school. The children especially were open and friendly, and their parents were kind too. With Tim in their midst, we thought there was a good chance the children would keep that openness towards disability well into adult life.

In his way, Tim has always been an ambassador for those who have physical and learning disabilities.

I remember that when I was a child, 'handicapped' children were not generally visible. They were not on my radar. Either they went to a special school – often residential – or they simply didn't leave home. As a result, I had grown up completely ignorant about disabilities. Handicap was an intimidating subject, the more so because it took place behind closed doors.

When we became parents to Tim, we both understood how essentially normal our son was. The medical labels were almost invisible to us. We always saw his real personality. We really liked that personality, and we completely loved our son. We saw that he had a right to an optimum life. We implicitly believed that he had a right to be included in society. And Tim, being a sociable soul, clearly agreed.

In Richmond, inclusion had sometimes been a challenge. But we quickly realised it was going to be more of a challenge in rural Wiltshire.

The school tried very hard, and their efforts were appreciated. I remember in particular one very considerate parent governor arranging a disabled parking bay right next to the school.

Socially though, it was very different to Richmond. It was a more homogenous society, and differences took longer for local people to adjust to. So there was never that sense of easy social life that we had enjoyed in Richmond. I missed that. I think Tim did too.

Tim did have lots of happy moments with his classmates. But I believe he found it harder to feel normal in a place where he wasn't considered normal. Over the next few years, he had a series of chest infections that impacted badly on his spinal curvature. During the time of the move he had also stopped seeing his osteopath, Sultana Khan. The gap probably did his health no favours.

We actually located Sultana again, funnily enough, living not that far from our new home. With the increased complexity of Tim's scoliosis, however, she felt he would be better off with an extremely experienced osteopath called Peter Cockhill, who runs a clinic called Stillpoint in Bath. Restarting osteopathy with Pete was one of the very best decisions we've made. Tim still has regular sessions to this day.

Tim did have a lovely teaching advisor who focused primarily on children with *physical* disabilities in mainstream schools. I don't think there was anyone who advised on complex *learning* disabilities in mainstream schools, because such children automatically went to a special school. In due course, the advisor started talking about visits to the local special school. We said we'd think about it.

We were aware that we were having different conversations about Tim's schooling than we'd had in Richmond. I felt regret, but it was time to let go and move on.

Growing family

One of the very best aspects about moving to Wiltshire was that we suddenly had more family members around, including my parents. Their support immediately made a difference to all of us. I'm sure they brought a real sense of security to Tim. He developed quite a thing about watching *Barney* videos in Grandma's kitchen, while eating cake and biscuits.

And then, just over a year after our arrival, Tim's little sister was born.

Steven and I had opted for a pregnancy with minimum intervention, and a home birth. We both knew that there was a higher than average risk of having a second baby with complications – especially as I would be 43 by the time she was born. Briefly, we had talked about it. We both felt strongly that our new baby would be loved and welcomed whatever. So we just went ahead with the pregnancy and I saw a midwife from time to time, and that was it.

Reality reminder: pregnancy is not a medical condition. It's a natural part of life.

Our decision took away so much anxiety. In its place, I experienced acceptance, and happiness. It was the sort of happiness that arrives when you let go of expectation and trust that whatever happens, all will be well.

One morning, late in the pregnancy, I woke up with a name on my lips: "Grace." It seemed like a beautiful name for anyone to be called. We didn't know that our baby was going to be a girl, but on another level, I did know. Steven liked the name Grace too. We didn't even bother to think of a boy's name.

Our baby was late. At around eight days late the midwife sent us to see a hospital consultant. When he heard about Tim he was astounded. "How is it possible that I haven't seen you before?" he said. So we explained our philosophy, and he was accepting of that. He saw no need for intervention, and nor did we.

In the end, our second baby arrived in her own good time, 11 days after her due date. She was born in our bed with no fewer than four midwives around us, due to a shift change and the presence of a student midwife.

When she emerged, she wasn't breathing. She was turning blue. A midwife gave her five puffs of oxygen, and then she started breathing. Somehow, we didn't doubt that she would be okay. It was clear that she was healthy, weighing in at 8 lb, 14 oz. I held her in my arms and looked down at her, absorbing the essence of this new individual. She was beautiful. "Hello, Grace, welcome to the world," I said gently, bathing her in love.

While our bedroom was efficiently cleaned up, Steven took her into Tim's empty room next door (Tim was at his grandparents' during the birth) and father lay down with baby daughter, bonding with her. Exhausted, I basked in happiness. I saw, intuitively, the four corners of our family – two parents, two children – and understood that each corner was equally part of the whole.

And life was good.

The Continuum Concept

For the first time, we experienced what it was like to have a child without complex needs – to be mainstream parents.

I breastfed our second baby exclusively for seven months. That wasn't a deliberate plan. I was simply letting her take to food in her own good time. Gradually, as she sat on my lap at the table, she started taking an interest in food, and I just fed her small bits from my plate. Then she began to have her own plate. She never had a single jar of commercial baby food.

The standard milestones that she reached astonished us. It was an absolute novelty when she started speaking, and having conversations with us. We also found, as she grew older, that she could be infinitely more demanding than her brother. We understood how lucky we had been, that Tim has always made it very easy for people to help him. Once I heard him say, subliminally, "People are very good at helping." I realised *this* was his world: one in which he accepts help. He trusts that help is available, and it generally is.

Having a second child changed the energy of the family. It created more scope for fun. Tim became a very happy audience to Grace's antics. In a way, it took the pressure off him. Now there were two children: each a unique individual, each free to be themselves.

There were challenges aplenty. The single hardest thing was having two children who couldn't walk. Can you imagine pushing one child in a wheelchair, and another younger child in a buggy? It's fine for those times when there are two adults around. But on a daily basis, it's just not feasible. There are double buggies you can get, but nothing that worked for our particular needs.

Luckily, I wasn't remotely interested in wheeling both my children around in a large, unwieldy vehicle. My outlook was very different.

Before Grace was born I had read *The Continuum Concept* by Jean Liedloff. This book had influenced me enormously. It made a lot of sense to me.

The Continuum Concept is based on observations of the author. She spent a period of time living with a tribe of Amazonian people. She noticed how contented the children were, compared with Western children. The same differences extended to the adults. It was a calm, happy society. She decided to work out why, and came up with the Continuum Concept.

The continuum is what we are biologically and epigenetically used to. For millennia, human babies were treated very differently to how we treat babies today.

In prehistory, babies were born when they were ready to be born. They were carried from the moment of birth, until they were ready to crawl or walk. They were fed breast milk when they wanted it, whenever they wanted it. They had constant body contact with an adult carer. They were never – *never* – left in a cot away from their mother. They were carried any which way over rough terrain. When they started crawling, they had no stair gates to protect them from dangerous drops. They had no special baby food. They had no nappies. Their carers tuned in pretty quickly to their toileting needs, sensing when a baby was about to empty its bladder and positioning them in a suitable place.

Jean Liedloff realised that all these factors together created happier babies, with a well-developed nervous system, and a good sense of their own safety and well-being.

I absorbed these lessons, and mourned the loss of natural upbringing in our own society. Then I proceeded to do what I could to let both Tim and Grace benefit from these ideas.

I blended Continuum with intuition, and basically began to listen to the needs of my children, without imposing too many external rules on them.

So Grace became a sling baby. Pushing Tim in his wheelchair suddenly became a whole lot easier when Grace was comfortably tucked up against my chest. She was as happy as anything – it was where she wanted to be. And Tim felt included on all our outings.

We had a blue tartan sling that was Grace's home and comfort zone. She watched the world from that sling: quiet and contented while her instincts to observe and learn were being met.

It was also easy to breastfeed Grace discreetly while she was in the sling. It just wasn't a big deal. It was rare that anyone even noticed. She was fed several times while standing in the supermarket queue. She was fed on a rare visit to church for a family event; in the cinema, in cafés….

One evening Steven and I went to a fundraising ball in Chippenham, our local town. I carried Grace, as usual, in the sling. She watched for a while, and then she fed, and slept. We bumped into other parents there who had had babies at the same time as Grace. Their babies had stayed at home with a babysitter. The parents were amazed that we could take Grace. They couldn't imagine their own baby behaving in that situation.

On more than one occasion I would be feeding Grace while a baby somewhere nearby would be crying loudly. The sound used to hurt me. I wanted that baby's evident needs to be met.

It's the norm in our society to ignore our babies' needs. Yet, at the same time, we dote on our infants. We create all sorts of structured activities for them, which often involve special clothes and equipment.

In the contented rainforest society that Jean Liedloff studied, parents didn't dote on their children. They loved them and treated them with respect, but they didn't let their lives revolve around the children. They let the children play, and let them join in with adult activities such as food preparation as and when they felt like it.

In the time span of humanity's life, we are just a heartbeat.

But in that heartbeat we have rejected so much of who we are, in favour of timetables and rules. We impose these on every new member of our society. We watch them deaden and become numb, just as we did at their age. We have disconnected with nature, and our own true nature.

As soon as Grace could toddle she would be in on the action, whatever it might be. I remember once hearing, subliminally, what seemed to be a core thought of hers: "If I can see everything, I will understand everything and I will be able to do everything."

She was a busy person, investigating everything. I remember one sunny day as I stood in the kitchen, I caught sight of a blonde thistledown head bobbing past the window outside. I could sense her contentment. It was one of those moments of sheer, carefree happiness.

We didn't overprotect her. For example, we decided not to put a stair gate up. I remember watching her at the top of the stairs, exploring the first steps. Like every Western parent, I felt an urge to say, "Be careful," to scoop her up and whisk her away from the precipice. But I didn't. I watched how carefully she explored, and how she learnt to climb down and up the stairs.

Outdoors, I noticed how she would follow my path exactly. She was learning how to negotiate obstacles by watching how the grown-ups did it.

We also gave her space to make mistakes.

Once, as a toddler, she was playing with a slightly older friend, Ben, in the garden. I was watching without interfering. I could see that she wasn't making her way around the garden as thoughtfully as usual. It seemed to me that she was 'showing off' in some way.

I watched her approach a pond. I observed her putting a foot over the green surface of the pond. I could see her thinking: "Is this solid ground? Can I walk on this?" She and I both knew we never walked over the bright green duckweed.

She put her foot over the duckweed, and she stepped on to it.

As I moved quickly towards her, she sank into the water, up to her chest. I could see her lips moving, and heard her say, "Oh." She was beginning to sway when I picked her out of the pond. She was covered in tiny bright green leaves. She was horrified, and began to wail. I took her indoors and cleaned her off.

My behaviour was unusual. But it wasn't dangerous. I was in tune with my young daughter. I could sense her mood changes with ease, and was alert to the change in her that day. Without shouting any warnings or interfering, I let Grace fall into the pond. But I knew it was something she would take care never to do again. And she didn't.

Tim continued at the local village school. A new headteacher turned up, who was warmly encouraging to Tim, and all the teachers welcomed Grace when she was born. But the Wild West saloon bar feeling never entirely disappeared. We both missed the social group we had had, and never quite found a replacement for it. Tim was happy and easy-going and enjoyed the company of the children in his class. He had a couple of brilliant and supportive teaching assistants, Naomi Irvine and Charis Higgs. But over time the invisible wall between him and the village school became more evident. He began to have sessions at the local special school. That, however, brought its own problems.

When Tim first went to the special school, he found it noisy, chaotic and very difficult. During the first year of visits, he became ill frequently with respiratory infections and his spinal curvature continued to worsen.

Gradually, he adapted. For several years he balanced the two schools. It seemed to be the best solution. He was a sociable soul who enjoyed being in a busy mainstream environment. At the same time, the special school provided him with more sensory teaching opportunities. Each school had some excellent teachers and assistants. Each school contained some lovely children.

He enjoyed the opportunities at each. But it continued to be a delicate balancing act. When he had a TA who was happy in the environment, things worked better.

At one point I was actively considering taking him out of the village school. He had a temporary TA who didn't seem to be thriving in the job, but wasn't admitting it. I really wondered if it would be better to move Tim. Steven got rather fed up with hearing me talking about the problems.

But then, I had a dream that changed my thinking.

Sometimes, the harder path is the right one

In the dream, I was standing outdoors on a dark and rainy night. I was holding a baby. The path ahead was flooded. It looked completely daunting. Although I wanted to take that route, I gave up and turned right to take another path.

But as I turned, I heard someone to the left, calling my name. I looked, and there, beyond the flooded section of the path, was the figure of a man. It was Christ.

He was beckoning me forward, through the floodwater. He indicated a simple rope, to my left, that had been erected at hand height. I put my hand on the rope, and walked forward, baby still in my arms. I walked through the floodwater, and it wasn't hard, although it didn't feel entirely safe. But I knew I would reach the dry land ahead. I was totally reassured by the figure of Christ.

When I woke up I felt strongly that the harder path – staying at the village school – was the right path. And after a while, things did get a little easier. Tim particularly loved the PE lessons, and being with the other children in the playground at break times. He actually continued to visit the village school for one or two sessions a week until the age of 12.

16. A narrow escape in Jacksonville

I'm going to tell you about Florida, 2010, when Tim became critically ill. He was 14. I want to tell you this story because it encapsulates the sense that he is, in some indefinable way, looked after. It also shows how premonitory dreams can help us be better prepared for life events, even if we don't understand them at the time. And it absolutely demonstrates the collective power of healing and prayer.

In the months leading up to this event, I had a series of premonitory dreams. A whole 18 months before, I dreamed that *we were all on a journey, travelling from our home in England. I whizzed ahead to an American hospital to sign forms – there was lots of paperwork. I was extremely happy.*

Of course, I didn't have a clue what this dream was about, but the happy feeling was clearly a good sign.

In another dream, *I was by the bedside of a young man who was very ill in hospital. I took a tube out of his mouth. He started talking in an American accent.*

Again, I couldn't begin to guess the meaning of this dream.

In the summer before the event, I dreamed that *we were touring an English hospital. It seemed old and tired, past its heyday. We met Tim's consultant. I asked her how she stayed current in her training. She replied, "Well, we do our best." I realised that I didn't want any member of my family to go there.*

This dream was easier to understand. I was feeling uneasy about our local hospital. Tim had been there on several occasions with chest infections. We'd encountered some very caring staff, and were truly grateful for the help that Tim had received. However, if there was a prize for the most dynamic, effective, visionary hospital... I don't think our local hospital at that time would have won it.

In the next dream, *the four of us were visiting a house where a rocket was about to go off. I helped Tim to get to the front, so he could see it. We knew when the rocket went off it would be BIG. Some kind of big, earth-shaking event was on its way.*

In between these dreams, waking life went on as normal. The messages of the dreams didn't seem to dovetail with what was happening right now in our lives. However, there was a subtle sense of something brewing, beneath the surface.

This would have been all too easy to miss, if the dreams hadn't been pointing out the same thing.

Steven was due to attend a conference in America, and suggested we go as a family. The conference was to be held on Amelia Island, in Florida.

I said, "Yes," straightaway. I noticed, however, that I had some mixed feelings. On the one hand, I wanted to go: it would be a great family holiday. On the other hand, there was something looming. It felt uncomfortable. I pushed it from my mind. I told myself that our son was in perfect health. There was nothing to worry about.

The bottom line is this: I said "yes" because I was immediately sure, without knowing why, that going to Florida at that time was the right thing to do.

The first week of our holiday seemed fine. During the second week, however, Tim began to look pale and tired. He began to develop a rash. Then, on the morning of Halloween, we discovered him lying motionless in his bed. His rash was far worse and he looked pale, almost blue. He was getting bluer. We knew something was very wrong.

We rushed to the local walk-in clinic where Tim was promptly given oxygen. Within 90 minutes, Tim and I had been transferred by ambulance to The Wolfson Children's Hospital in nearby Jacksonville. Steven and Grace cleared our room, checked out of the hotel, and followed by car. We were told that Tim had a dangerous illness, called varicella pneumonia – a complication of chicken pox. A rash covered his body and, more dangerously, the inner surfaces of his lungs. The prognosis was extremely poor.

I think it must have felt to Tim as though his lungs and entire body were on fire.

Varicella pneumonia, I read later, has a mortality rate of 50%. For Tim, with his severe scoliosis, we were told, kindly but frankly, that there was next to no hope. "I'm amazed he's still alive," said Dr Benjamin-Thorpe who admitted him to PICU, the Pediatric Intensive Care Unit. However, she also made it clear that the team would do whatever they could to get him through.

"We understand that you believe there's very little chance of him getting through this," we told her. "But you don't know Tim. If anyone can get through it, he can."

By the early evening, the decision was made to put Tim on a ventilator – a machine that would do his breathing for him. We were told that there was a risk of cardiac arrest without intubation. We were told that intubation was the act of inserting a tube into his trachea, or windpipe, to keep it open and deliver mechanized, oxygen-rich air flow. We were told – and it was obvious – that his lungs were taking in less and less oxygen, that he wouldn't survive without this intervention.

We listened to this in a state of shock. It felt that we were living a nightmare. This was new territory for us. Although Timmy had had many chest infections, they had not been anywhere near this severe.

While he was being intubated, Steven, Grace and I went to the family room just outside the ward. It was empty, apart from the three of us. We stood together, hugging. I said a prayer for all of us, and it went along these lines.

"Dear God," I said. "Thank you for the wonderful presence of Tim in our lives. Thank you for all that he has brought to us. We love him so much. We're so sorry that he's in such pain now. Thank you for bringing us to this hospital, with its amazing team of people who can help him.

"With all our hearts, we want Tim well again. Please make him well again, if that is for his highest good. But more than anything, we want whatever's best for him. We hand him over to you now, dear God. We entrust him to you."

We knew, somehow, that it was important to let go. We gave him unconditional love and blessing. We gave the whole medical team unconditional love and blessing. And we trusted.

Tim was placed in a quarantined room. We had to wear gowns, masks and gloves to enter it. The next day, a consultant told us that a child with no underlying health issues might remain on a ventilator for six days, and take a further nine months to recover completely. "In your son's case," he said, stretching his arms out as wide as he could, "you could stretch that time scale out as long as you like."

He also told us that Tim would be unable to return to England for a very long time, and we might want to think about more long-term accommodation for ourselves in America.

The medical staff still didn't really believe that he would make it, though they did their very best and they hoped.

Tim spent six days, in a medically induced coma, on a ventilator. A total of 13 tubes entered his body during that time, carrying a complex mixture of medication and nutrition. I requested that probiotics be added to the liquid food, to help counteract the effect of antibiotics. And I was favourably surprised when this was quickly done. The nurses were keen to explain that the value of probiotics was recognised by the medical team.

I also spoke to Tim's local homeopath, Chris Fixsen, in Wiltshire and we arranged for Tim to receive a remedy every day. This was administered as a drop on the lips. I insisted on doing this with the consultants' knowledge and consent.

During the six days, Tim had episodes in which his oxygen levels plummeted. I was with him night and day, apart from regular periods when Steven took over. Grace was also with us for the entire period, although she spent much briefer periods in Tim's room. Seeing her, aged six, gowned-up with mask and gloves to visit her older brother was a bitter-sweet experience.

It was of course a very intense period. We had no idea whether Tim would survive.

Our world was a pale and swollen son in a high-tech bed that weighed him at regular intervals. Our world was bleeping machines. Our world was a window of sky, and a larger picture window overlooking the central unit.

My world was the silent and steady practice of unobtrusively giving Tim healing, punctuated by numerous visits and constant alarms, both Tim's and other children's in their own glass rooms.

Our world was daily phone calls from Steven's parents, and my parents, and numerous texts, calls and other support from our families and friends.

My world was a long orange dress that I used as a nightgown, and two loose blue tops with cropped trousers that I wore during the day. We had overstayed our holiday and the weather had turned. I hadn't packed for Florida in November.

It seemed to me that there was something monastic about keeping watch over a loved one in care. Tim's extreme danger meant that my mind was fully present. I wasn't distracted. The normal diversions with which we fill our lives held no interest for me. The single issue that fully engaged me was Tim's health.

There was also room to worry about his sister. But she was spending a lot of time with her dad, and seemed to cope by having an unquenchable belief that Tim would pull through. She was also receiving presents from well-wishers every day. "I wonder what I'll receive today," she would say, with great anticipation. And sure enough, she would receive something: a doll, a game, a book, some drawing materials, and another doll....

We were overwhelmed by the support we received within the hospital. The consultant in charge during this period was Dr Kevin Sullivan, a one-time New York firefighter who now fought for the lives of the children in his care with absolute conviction and energy. We felt he was the ideal person to have on Tim's side.

I wrote in my blog at the time:

The medical team in PICU, Wolfson Children's Hospital has been brilliant, absolutely brilliant. The medical resources are state of the art. And the whole place is supported by a huge, enthusiastic network of benefactors and volunteers, whose influence is everywhere.

Strangers have hugged us like old family friends, and prayed for our son. Our children have been showered with presents, attention and care. We've been given a family room at the local Ronald McDonald House, a sanctuary where delicious evening meals are donated and cooked for us and the other families staying there. Child-friendly activities are organised – this evening it was gingerbread house decorating, with story.

One of the most heart-warming aspects of that post was that some of the hospital staff responded online with appreciative comments. These included Dr Benjamin-Thorpe, the immensely able doctor who had admitted Tim; Misty Weise, one of the wonderful team of nurses who cared for him; and Katie Wassil, one of the dedicated pharmacists who prepared his complex medication. The blog post also included lots of warmly supportive comments from Tim's grandma, Barbara, now living in Ireland, along with Tim's granddad John.

One day I visited the hospital chapel, and meditated with a couple of others, both members of staff, I think, who also turned up. Other times, I went to the Friends' library, and borrowed healing music that I played endlessly to our sleeping son. Some days Steven, Grace and I went to a little café in the hospital where you could sit outside, by St Johns River, and watch wild dolphins swimming in the deep middle parts of the wide water. We were thrilled to see these and took them to be a sign of healing.

I happened to have a copy of a prayer with me, by Lorna Byrne. It came from her book, *Angels in My Hair*. Every evening I would read this prayer aloud, beside our sleeping son. I loved the sense of quiet reassurance it gave me. It helped me to let go, and trust that a higher power was helping Tim, in ways that were beyond my imagining. Even when I look at this prayer today, it has a similar, reassuring effect. I reproduce it here with the kind permission of Lorna Byrne, who sent me a message saying that this prayer is meant for sharing. She also mentioned that it is meant to be written *exactly* as I show it below.

Prayer of Thy Healing Angels
That is carried from God by Michael, Thy Archangel

Pour out, Thy Healing Angels,
Thy Heavenly Host upon me,
And upon those that I love,
Let me feel the beam of Thy
Healing Angels upon me,
The light of Your Healing Hands.
I will let Thy Healing begin,
Whatever way God grants it,
Amen.

We also asked my photographer father to send some pictures from home, that we could put up in Tim's room, to bring the energy of home, the *sanctuary* of home, to his bedside. Some of the photos were flowers from the garden. Some were pictures of us and other family members.

Among the photos was one of the four of us, waving from windows in our old stone house. That amazed the medical staff, as it looked so different from the houses of Jacksonville. "It's like something out of a fairy tale, or a movie," was one comment.

Periodically, Tim would have 'an episode'. His oxygen

saturation levels would slide rapidly downwards. Medical staff would cluster around his bed, doing whatever they could to encourage his oxygen levels to improve. Steven would also stand by the bed, willing our son to recover.

Sometimes, during these episodes, I would stand by Tim's bed, but other times I was drawn to sit quietly in a chair in a corner of the room. There I would focus on being still while all the activity and emergency went around me. I held the moment in my heart. Helped by the regular meditation that I did, and still do, I went into a different space. It was as if I tuned into a radio frequency of relative calmness and well-being. Within this space it seemed to me that I held Tim, and the whole situation, in waves of light and love.

At these times, it appeared to me as though time and space became altered – as if I could actually see another picture of the ward, which overlaid my vision like a translucent envelope. In this way I saw, in my mind's eye, that Tim was lying on a huge cushion of white light – strands of light. The strands seemed to come from many different directions. I understood that many strands of light came from hundreds of people praying in Britain, Ireland and America. I also understood that much of the light came from another dimension that wasn't visible to me.

But then during one of Tim's episodes, that other dimension *did* become visible, albeit still with a transparency to it. It seemed to me that I saw figures: tall, elongated, slender and flowing. They had an air of compassion, purpose and capability. These figures were mainly beyond the humans clustered around his bed, but some were among them. I felt there was, as it were, a celestial medical team that was also working on Tim, helping the human staff. It seemed as though the figures themselves were made of white light.

They reminded me strongly of the team of healing figures that I've mentioned before: the ones I saw in a dream, a few months after Tim was born. Seeing them again filled me with reassurance and hope.

Among the beings of light, in the foreground, was a celestial figure who *was* dominant. He – I shall say he – was standing to the left of Tim's bed as I was looking at it. This figure was tall, and broader than the others. He held a sword vertically downwards. The handle of the sword was at his chest height. The tip was resting on the floor, at his feet.

When I saw this figure, I felt immediately reassured. To be accurate, I was still frightened. I remained frightened during the whole time Tim was in intensive care. But along with the fear, I felt certain that Tim would get through his illness. The figure looked, to my perception at that time, like the Archangel Michael. I felt he was there to protect Tim and keep him safe. There was a solidity to him that felt different to the members of the celestial healing team. There was a huge, fierce and strong sense of reassurance and protection emanating from him.

At this point, Tim's oxygen levels shot up again, and the humans in the room visibly relaxed. Steven turned to me. My perspective shifted. I could no longer see the celestial world.

"Are you okay?" he asked.

"Yes, I'm okay," I answered. I could find no words to explain my experience. I knew how strange it would sound, so I said nothing about it.

Rocky road

Although the doctors kept urging us not to expect too much, Tim made good progress. His 'episodes' gradually became less severe. Often I would simply stand by him and talk to him gently, telling him how well the air was entering him and bringing him the wonderful oxygen he needed, and removing the carbon dioxide he no longer required, and that he was getting better with every breath. I used a similar tone to the one I use in guided meditations with my clients. One of the nurses told me that word had got around that I could "talk his sats up" – I could encourage him to become better oxygenated through the gentle words. Of course, the next time I tried it, in front of a nurse, I felt very self-conscious and nothing particularly seemed to happen. But then I got over the self-consciousness and continued the practice anyway. It was just in my nature to do it.

After six days, Tim's sedation was reduced. He was taken off the ventilator and given a BiPAP mask, a less invasive way of directing oxygen at pressure into the lungs. That morning contained hope and fear in almost equal measures. As he gained consciousness, he was clearly very uncomfortable with the BiPAP. The high-pressure mask inhaled for him, at a pace that he could not control.

Two kind and supportive relatives of Steven's, Helen and Joe LoTruglio, turned up on that morning – they were living further south along the Florida coast at the time. They must have been quietly shocked to see Tim showing signs of distress as he gradually regained consciousness. His oxygen levels were erratic. Although it was a good sign that Tim had come off the ventilator, nobody knew whether he would be able to breathe well enough with the BiPAP.

Helen and Joe took Grace out, which she loved. By the end of that day, Tim was more settled and we were cautiously hopeful. The next day both Grace and I went out with Helen and Joe, at Steven's insistence while he sat with Tim. Steven felt I needed to get out of PICU. It was probably a good idea. It certainly made a huge difference that Helen and Joe gave their support to all of us during that time, when we were far from home.

Day after day, Tim continued to improve. His rate of recovery was, given his underlying health issues, miraculous.

One morning the doctors, headed by Dr Sullivan, were doing their usual round. They stopped outside his cubicle to discuss his case. I joined them. Suddenly, Dr Sullivan stopped talking. I realised that everyone was staring into Tim's cubicle. And there, from the bed, Tim's head was raised and he was staring back. He was indisputably observing them all, assessing them.

The medical team was thrilled. They all waved to him and smiled, and talked to him through the glass. It was the first time they had really seen Tim, the person. And I could tell that they were registering Tim's innate brightness, as well as his evident improvement.

Later that day, I heard Dr Sullivan talking on the phone to Tim's insurers (luckily Tim had full medical insurance). "He's high-functioning microcephalic," he was saying. I felt obscurely pleased. High-functioning seemed a fine thing to be, whatever medical label it was attached to.

Dr Sullivan got Tim's measure straight away. He spotted that Tim was "eyeballing" the spaghetti of tubes that were still connecting Tim to various medicines and equipment. "Anything he wasn't born with, he'll pull out," said Dr Sullivan, and he ensured that the tubes were removed from Tim as quickly as possible.

Tim continued to improve. And, just 17 days after admittance, he flew back to England in an air ambulance, a Learjet. He was still receiving oxygen through a small mask. I travelled with him, over the vast expanses of Canada, over the breathtakingly beautiful, snowy landscape of Greenland, and over the rainy, grey landscape of Iceland. In each country we stopped at a bleak, cold airfield for a fuelling and comfort stop. There were no toilets on the plane!

Meanwhile, Steven and Grace flew back with BA. That company had kindly kept our return tickets open when Tim became ill and we had to forgo our scheduled flight home. Gestures like that added to our collective feeling of gratitude.

By the time the Learjet had landed in Bristol, Tim needed no more supplementary oxygen. He spent one night in hospital in Bath, as a precaution. Then he came home, back to our lovely welcoming old stone house in Wiltshire.

A few weeks later Tim had a routine medical check-up with

a consultant. "You were very lucky," said the consultant. "I think if you'd been in England, it might have been a different outcome." It was something said quietly, in passing, that would never be repeated by that individual again. But I heard it, and I record it now.

Tim would take around nine months to get over his illness. In all respects, his rate of recovery was like that of a child without lung and health issues, as had been described by the consultant on the morning after Tim was admitted to Intensive Care. His journey back to health was simply amazing.

But he was to face one more challenge during that recovery period.

Goodbye, Dr Nocebo

The following Easter, Tim was still convalescing after his critical illness in Florida. We were back in England, and he had caught a new chest infection. He went to hospital where he was put on intravenous antibiotics. I stayed with him.

We sat in the hospital, day after day, and nothing much seemed to be happening. Tim wasn't getting worse, but he wasn't getting better either. Some days we didn't even spot a doctor. Tim was scarcely eating, so I asked to see a nutritionist. I was told that all the paediatric ones were away. After a couple of days, an adult one materialised and gave me some food supplements. I was grateful for those, but surprised that I had to work so hard to get them. Surely this was the sort of thing that Tim's doctors should pick up on?

To be fair, there were some very good nurses around, and a lovely schoolteacher too. But apart from them, the atmosphere seemed lacklustre. I couldn't help comparing it with the medical team that had saved Tim's life in Florida. *They* had seemed full of energy and a belief in their medicine. They didn't think Tim would pull through, but they did everything in their power to help him, and were thrilled when he made it.

Yet now, in England, it felt as though Tim had been somehow written off.

One morning a doctor came into Tim's ward. It wouldn't be fair to give his real name, so I shall call him Dr Nocebo.

Absolutely, the name is symbolic.

The nocebo effect got a dishonourable mention earlier in my story. It's a widely described phenomenon that is activated when a person in a position of authority, such as a doctor, leads another to believe that they are going to get worse. This harnesses, in a negative way, the body's own power to alter health outcomes. If, as so often happens, the patient believes the doctor, the nocebo prediction can become a self-fulfilling prophecy.

The opposite of the nocebo effect is the better-known placebo effect. Drug trials always have to take the placebo effect into account because a high percentage of recipients of the inactive control medication will get better – due to their belief in an imaginary medicine. Drug companies dismiss this as an annoying anomaly. But actually, it's an indication that healing can happen spontaneously when the right conditions of belief are in place.

Unfortunately for us, it was Dr Nocebo who walked into Tim's ward that morning. On this occasion, the doctor of doom was accompanied by a handful of medical students.

Dr Nocebo gave Tim a cursory examination. He noticed Tim's physical disabilities: his severe scoliosis, his tendency to lie still while he's ill.

Then he turned to me and told me, in graphic detail, how Tim was going to get more and more chest infections and they would become more and more frequent. And he would die – the implication was sooner rather than later.

As he talked, I felt faint. There was something inhuman about the way Dr Nocebo was delivering his damning news. It almost felt as though he was showing off his power in front of his students.

That evening, I went to a small parents' bedroom near the

ward. I got into bed. I lay there, in the dark, and worried about Tim's slow rate of recovery.

And then it happened. I heard a voice: loudly, insistently, inside my mind.

"Suzanne," it said. That was all. But accompanying my name came all sorts of information. It was a full conversation, delivered in one word.

I realised straight away that I had fallen prey to the nocebo effect on my son's behalf. I had been picturing Tim getting more and more poorly. I had believed Dr Nocebo's words.

I now had an urgent job to do. I needed to visualise my son well. And I needed to keep doing it.

The actual visualisation came with great ease. It was as if someone were leading me through it.

First I pictured, in great detail, that I was standing in beautiful countryside. There were fruit trees in blossom all around. In front of me was a healing temple. I walked up ten steps, and entered the temple. I went to the reception desk, and signed in. I was given a special disc to wear around my neck, over my heart.

I walked across the light and airy atrium, to the healing space at the heart of the temple. There, I took a seat. In front of me was a shimmering space. I pictured Tim in the space, receiving all the healing he required. Before my eyes, he became well and strong.

I left the temple, still wearing the disc.

The next day, Steven was the lucky one who got to see Dr Nocebo. The doctor of doom duly gave Steven the same talk he gave me: your son will soon die, etc.

Steven, being the practical one, asked: "Yes, but what about exercise? Won't that help?"

Steven was fully aware that Tim normally does lots of physiotherapy and yoga. Dr Nocebo just saw a pale and poorly disabled teenager. He had no idea that when Tim is well he can be reasonably active. He can walk up and down stairs with support. He can even stand up on one leg, with support, and do the Tree position in yoga.

Take that, Dr Nocebo!

"Oh yes," said Dr Nocebo, surprised. "Yes, that could help."

In my imagination, I returned to the temple once a day. Each time, I first went to the reception desk. My disc was checked. Each time it was black and smoky with negative energy. It felt polluted. So I handed it in and received a new one. And then I went to the healing space in the heart of the temple, and pictured Tim strong and well.

In real life, Tim got better, and we left the hospital. But even at home, whenever I felt the need, I continued to visit the healing temple, in my imagination, on his behalf.

I noticed, on my visits, that the discs weren't getting so polluted. Then, on one visit, I was given a more permanent healing disc to wear. It was gold and iridescent: beautiful. People gathered round to congratulate me. I realised that I had graduated to a new level.

The new disc was designed to stay naturally clean of negative pollution. However, I understood that it would still be wise to get the healing disc checked at the reception desk from time to time.

Soon after Tim's encounter with Dr Nocebo, I realised that there was just one more thing to do: we needed to change hospitals. So I arranged for Tim's care to be transferred to a newer and better hospital. We didn't get to see the new consultant for 18 months though. There was no need. Despite his disabilities, Tim enjoyed a period of excellent health.

Unfortunately, Dr Nocebo has many cousins, all equally negative and miserable. So if you happen to encounter one of them, remember this: when Dr (or Mr or Ms) Nocebo talks negative, it's up to you to visualise positive.

17. Integration

I'm going to tell you something now that I haven't shared with too many people.

Just before I left boarding school, when I was 18, I had an out-of-body experience that scared me. It was night. I was sleeping in a single dorm. Without warning, I found myself floating high up in the room. I was at right angles to my body. I could see my body lying on the bed. I was floating by the top of the window.

At the other end of the room, roughly where the door would be, but higher, stood a tall figure. He was partially in darkness. He was not frightening in himself, but I was frightened to see him. Although I wasn't religious, I was raised in a Christian culture: I saw him as Christ.

He said one word to me:

"Come."

As soon as he said that, I became aware of a tunnel of light to his left, and my right, leading upwards, diagonally out of the room. There was a sound emanating from the tunnel; it seemed to come from the walls of the tunnel itself, although the tunnel didn't have walls as such. It was more like a vortex. It felt as though the walls were made out of sound, and light.

I couldn't tell you exactly what the sound was. It seemed to have many tones within it. I interpreted it as countless angels singing.

I was frightened. I thought maybe I was dying or, even, being invited to die. I knew that I wanted to live.

I replied, in my mind:

"Not yet, it's not my time."

And with those words, everything vanished. I was back in my body, touching my body and checking that it and I were still in the physical realm.

The next morning I moved out of the single dorm. I swapped

places with a girl who was in a double dorm next door to mine. I just knew that I didn't want to be on my own at night.

Here's the thing. If we are not open to the message, it will be sent through another channel. Two nights after my out-of-body experience, I had a most amazing dream. It was the sort of dream you remember for your whole life. It was clearly a form of guidance, although it would be decades before the meaning became clear.

This was the dream.

Inside the mountain, many choices

I am 18. I live inside a mountain, along with everyone I have ever known. Where you live depends upon your family's occupation. That's the way it's always been. I've never questioned it. Why would I? My parents are drapers, so we live on Drapers' Street. The shopfronts are full of different coloured fabrics.

There is a particular atmosphere in our street. It's hard for me to explain, as it's what I've always known. It's familiar. It's home. I think our family has always lived here, back through many generations. We have breathed in the scent of fabric all our lives.

In the mountain we never see natural light. We are used to artificial lamps. Despite this, there is one real, live tree that grows not far from where we live. It's in the centre of town, in an open space. The tree is a large, old weeping willow. It's beautiful, really special.

I am in my final school year. I will be leaving very soon, as will all my classmates. This evening there will be a leaver's party at the willow tree. We're all excited.

I choose my clothes: a periwinkle blue shift dress, with a silver belt. I tie a silver scarf in my hair. I go to the tree with my friends and we dance, and have enormous fun.

The next day, we get the Tour.

The Tour is designed to broaden our minds and show us the

diversity of life in our world. We travel with our teachers in small groups to different parts of the mountain. We explore a wide variety of regions, all hewn out of the rock that contains us. First of all, we visit a number of streets. These are like Drapers Street, but each is different in its own particular way. Some of these are of course already familiar to us.

But then we walk further, away from the centre... towards, someone whispers, the edge of the mountain.

In these areas there are no streets, just narrow passages that open out into large rooms, or chambers.

The rock in the passageways often looks roughly hewn. You can tell you're not in the centre. It's all much more primitive looking. It looks ancient. I think this is where our earliest ancestors lived.

We go through one narrow passage that opens out into a huge, rather grandiose chamber. Inside the chamber there are many beautiful people. The women are wearing elaborate pastel silk ball gowns. The men are in satin breeches and jackets.

The beautiful people are promenading. Some are dancing. Quite a few are gazing at themselves in mirrors. We gaze back at them in awe.

"Look carefully," says our teacher.

And then we notice that the beautiful people are somehow hollow inside. Although they are living and moving, they appear to have no heart. When I realise that, I feel my stomach lurch. There is something rather unpleasant about the beautiful people, even though they look so attractive.

We continue our journey and walk along another narrow passage. It's so narrow; I find it hard to breathe. Then the passage opens out into another huge chamber. This one, however, is not grandiose. It is humble in the extreme. The people here are all disabled. Some cannot walk, and are in wheelchairs. Others can walk, but their bodies don't work properly.

I am shocked at seeing all these disabled people. I'm not used to seeing anyone like this. They must all live here, I think.

"Look carefully," says our teacher, again.

And then we notice that the hearts of the disabled people are gorgeous and glowing. They are beautiful on the inside, and that beauty shines outwards from their centre.

Our teacher directs us to leave the chamber of disabled people. I confess I am rather glad. Even though they have warm hearts, it's unsettling to witness their disabilities.

We continue to move outwards from the centre, towards the edge of the mountain. We have to walk along an extremely narrow passage. I don't like this at all. I feel claustrophobic. Then, thankfully, we squeeze through and find ourselves in yet another enormous chamber.

This one is empty.

Correction: the chamber is empty, but the floor is covered in ice.

I am given a pair of ice skates, and I fasten them on. Then I glide out on to the ice.

I am so happy.

There is space. There is freedom.

This is what it's all about, I say to myself. This is why we are here.

And I skate on with absolute, effortless joy.

As soon as I woke up, I wrote an account of that dream. I shared it with a couple of friends. Then I put it away.

After I left school, I spent three years at the University of Cambridge. Then I went to London and worked on several glossy magazines. The cover models were photoshopped to look flawless. I remember the first time I saw young models come into the editorial offices with their portfolios. I was struck by how thin they were. Compared with their covers, they lacked radiance. I wondered at the process that turned these less than glowing girls into perfect examples of female beauty.

And so, I entered the chamber of the beautiful, yet hollow, people.

When I was 35, I gave birth to a baby boy with complex and visible disabilities. He was unusually thin and wiry. Doctors described his features as 'dysmorphic'. That's just another way of saying misshapen. But I thought he was beautiful. I could see how gorgeous he was on the inside, as well as on the outside. His inner beauty made him glow.

And so, I entered the chamber of the disabled people who were beautiful on the inside (and out).

A few years after Tim was born, I found my record of the Mountain dream. I was shocked to discover that I had omitted any mention of the disabled people. And yet I remembered them vividly. They were a central component of the dream.

It was an insight into how we humans can become unconscious of things we can't handle. What else, I wondered, am I unconscious of? That question fuelled the next stage of my career.

Over the following years, I retrained. I became a spiritual healer. I wrote a book supporting the interests of children with special needs, and their families. In my work, I tried to use the skills I had learned at Cambridge, and in London, and apply them to the world of cognitive and physical disabilities. I understood that we are all normal. We are all intelligent. We are all beautiful. We all have our own individual style. We all deserve to live a meaningful life.

And so, I entered the chamber of ice. On the ice I could move with effortless joy, because I was accepting all aspects of who I was, of what humanity was. I was therefore truly being myself.

The chamber of ice has a personal meaning for me, one that you would never find in a dream dictionary.

That's why I believe the best dream dictionaries are the ones we write ourselves.

Here is the personal meaning....

During my two years of childhood in Russia, I used to go ice-skating with my family in the winter. My younger brother became rather good at ice-skating and adopted a catchphrase. He used this whenever he found he had mastered some new talent. "It's so easy, I could do it on ice," he'd say. Over time the catchphrase became shorter:

"I could do it on ice."

Every new talent can be a bit like that, I suspect. We have to practise, and keep practising. It's such hard work. It's like walking a narrow tunnel where we just have to keep pushing on. It can get rather joyless (though it doesn't have to). We think a hundred times that we'll never master this new talent. And then, one day, we do. It's as if the narrow tunnel of hard work and relentless practice has opened out into a new world of fun and possibility. The new talent has become so easy we could do it on ice.

Every new mindset is like that too. It takes time to assimilate new ideas and integrate them into our lives.

There is a rather lovely postscript to this story. Last winter Steven and I decided to go ice-skating with both our children. When we got to the rink in Swindon, we discovered that ramps are provided for wheelchair users to go directly on to the ice. So Steven, Tim, Grace and I all got on the ice and skated around. Tim in his chair actually provided a steady support to the rest of us. And for a while, the four of us held hands, or wheelchair handles, while we skated together over the ice.

That will be one of my lifelong happy memories: four people hand in hand, hands on handles, gliding over the ice.

Tim continues his amazing journey. He continues being an unofficial ambassador for disabilities. Wherever Tim goes, ripples appear in the air around him. People notice him, and are changed, one way or another. We saw this most recently on a family holiday to Hong Kong.

In an Asian society where people with cognitive and physical disabilities have traditionally been kept away from the public eye, accompanied by a sense of shame, the sight of Tim being a valued member of our family, out to look at the views and eat in nice restaurants, was always going to create ripples. We could have felt embarrassed as a family, but we didn't. Our previous adventures – all the events outlined in this book – had given us confidence. In some unspoken but significant way, we understood that we were there to see – and be seen.

Hopefully the changes created in the air around Tim are for the better.

Recently, Tim turned 18, and is now officially an adult. So I guess that means he is no longer a Miracle Child. He must now be a Miracle Adult.

To celebrate, he had a big lunch party at Bowood, a nearby hotel. The theme was elephants (one of his favourite animals). Lots of lovely, supportive friends and family turned up. There was a giant blue cardboard elephant, painted by all the family, which we'd turned into a postbox. Instead of bringing gifts, people put donations into the elephant postbox. The funds received went to Tim's school, and also to an Asian elephant charity. Tim has never been interested in lots of possessions. But he does love a good atmosphere. And the atmosphere of giving to good causes was one that suited him well.

I need to say this single, important fact: we feel so thrilled that after all his challenges, Tim has made it to adulthood.

The challenges aren't over. But we do believe in celebrating the small steps. And making it to adulthood is actually a pretty big step.

We are hoping that when he leaves school, in a few months' time, he will be able to attend National Star, an outstanding college near Cheltenham for differently abled people. That will give him exciting new opportunities for further progress and independence.

Remember to fight

There's something else that Tim would like me to say. I was talking with some relatives about Tim's Florida experience, just yesterday. I was describing how we felt we had to let go and trust that the medical team would save Tim. When I said this, Tim let out a huge, angry cry – not something he often does. He was clearly agitated.

"Have I got it wrong, Tim?" I asked him. "Is it not about letting go? Do you actually need to be really determined and fight to get well?"

Tim quietened at once and signed a simple, "Yes."

So let's put the record straight. Tim wanted to get well. He was determined to get well. And he did everything in his power to recover.

He's had that determination all his life. It has helped him immeasurably.

Creating quiet space

Nowadays, apart from the occasional social event, I do actively choose a quiet life. It's an absolute necessity for me. I love giving time each day to the richness and guidance of inner thoughts. It astonishes me how little this is valued or even understood in our society.

Unfortunately, I can be as guilty of this as anyone.

Even though I value the inner world, my actions do not always reflect this. All too often, I find myself squeezing ten minutes of meditation between activities. Many times when I'm rushing through my life I just stop on the side of the road – ancient Silbury Hill near Avebury Stone Circle is a favourite place not far from where I live – and allow myself a few quiet minutes.

I am convinced that these quiet moments create ripples within and around each one of us. We become calmer, happier people. We spread that calm into the world. We spread it in our immediate vicinity. And also, as we are all connected, we spread it holographically into the universe. And the universe ripples back to us, with myriad spiritual insights that are refreshing and illuminating.

My spiritual practice includes meditation, gentle stretches, and affirmations. Here is an affirmation that I have repeated over many years:

> *I love and accept myself as I am.*
> *I forgive myself everything.*
> *I love and accept myself as I am.*
> *I forgive everybody everything.*

I also appreciate the peace and safety that I experience when I say:

> *I am safe, and all is well.*

And I feel uplifted when I make a point of appreciating my life:

> *I give thanks for this day, and all that it contains.*
> *I bless this day with love and gratitude.*

Thank you for reading our story. You are a unique being, on your own unique path. Your journey will be different from ours, but there will be parallels along the way. I hope you know that you are a loveable and wonderful person, doing the very best you can, at every point. I hope you forgive yourself everything. And I hope you understand that while you are the very best expert in your own life, your wisdom comes from the same divine source that breathes life into all of us. Your best way of accessing that wisdom is to relax. Let it enter you.

> *We are safe, and all is well.*

I wish you love and happiness in your own life, now and always.

Appendix

Poppy Exercise: love and blessing

This meditation is helpful for increasing your sense of open-hearted compassion for all living beings.

Imagine that you are standing, or sitting, in a beautiful poppy field in a natural landscape. Vibrant red flowers are swaying on long green stems all around you. Somewhere nearby, a small river is running lazily by. It flows under a stone bridge, on its way through the field and on to the distant sea.

You are aware of a road in the distance, with the 'swish, swish' of cars passing.

Here, in the field, it's incredibly peaceful, and beautiful. There are some small birds swooping through the air, singing their songs.

You are surrounded by green and red: a field of green leaves, with the red of countless poppies, bobbing on top of the green. Above it all is the blue, blue sky. It is incredibly peaceful.

A breeze flows through the field, gently ruffling the poppies, gently brushing against your skin and your hair.

The sun shines warmly down, touching the top of your head. You feel safe here, and loved.

And now, simply imagine that every poppy in the field represents a human being – a human soul.

As you stand, or sit in the field, say these following words in your mind:

To all in front of me, I love you and bless you.
To all behind me, I love you and bless you.
To all to my right, I love you and bless you.
To all to my left, I love you and bless you.
To all above me, I love you and bless you.
To all below me, I love you and bless you.

To me myself, I love me and bless me.

As you say these words, cultivate a feeling of love and compassion to all living beings.

The more you practise this meditation, the easier it becomes. It's good to do this every day at the beginning. Less often is fine later on, as its energy becomes integrated within you.

Over time, you may find that you no longer visualise the poppy field. Instead, you visualise human beings directly: all those who are in front, behind, and so on.

Over time, this meditation can help you to become less judgmental (most of us are a little judgmental, at least some of the time). It can help you feel open-hearted to all people. It can improve all your relationships, including your relationship with yourself.

It is common for people who walk this path to find that they encounter fewer 'difficult' people.

The reason for this is simple. The poppy field meditation helps you to be forgiving and unconditionally loving. That cleans up your inner world immeasurably.

As you clean up your inner world, your outer world cleans up too.

Over time, you find your outer world muddies up again. It may be that more difficult people enter your life. If that happens, simply picture yourself in the poppy field again.

The poppy field reminds us that we are all beautiful human souls: all living, and growing, and trying our very best.

It reminds us that we ourselves are loved.

It reminds us that all are loved.

A note to the reader

Thank you for reading *This One is Special*. If you have gained as much from reading it as I have in writing it, then I am extremely happy. If you feel drawn to, please feel free to add your review of the book to your favourite online site for feedback. Also, if you'd like to read more of my writings or connect through social media, please visit my website:
suzanneaskham.com
You can also follow our son Tim on
instagram.com/timaskhamday
Warm wishes, Suzanne

BOOKS

O-BOOKS

SPIRITUALITY

O is a symbol of the world, of oneness and unity; this eye
represents knowledge and insight. We publish titles on general
spirituality and living a spiritual life. We aim to inform and
help you on your own journey in this life.
If you have enjoyed this book, why not tell other readers by
posting a review on your preferred book site?

Recent bestsellers from O-Books are:

Heart of Tantric Sex
Diana Richardson
Revealing Eastern secrets of deep love and intimacy to Western couples.
Paperback: 978-1-90381-637-0 ebook: 978-1-84694-637-0

Crystal Prescriptions
The A-Z guide to over 1,200 symptoms and their healing crystals
Judy Hall
The first in the popular series of six books, this handy little guide is packed as tight as a pill-bottle with crystal remedies for ailments.
Paperback: 978-1-90504-740-6 ebook: 978-1-84694-629-5

Take Me To Truth
Undoing the Ego
Nouk Sanchez, Tomas Vieira
The best-selling step-by-step book on shedding the Ego, using the teachings of *A Course In Miracles*.
Paperback: 978-1-84694-050-7 ebook: 978-1-84694-654-7

The 7 Myths about Love...Actually!
The journey from your HEAD to the HEART of your SOUL
Mike George
Smashes all the myths about LOVE.
Paperback: 978-1-84694-288-4 ebook: 978-1-84694-682-0

The Holy Spirit's Interpretation of the New Testament
A course in Understanding and Acceptance
Regina Dawn Akers
Following on from the strength of *A Course In Miracles*, NTI
teaches us how to experience the love and oneness of God.
Paperback: 978-1-84694-085-9 ebook: 978-1-78099-083-5

The Message of A Course In Miracles
A translation of the text in plain language
Elizabeth A. Cronkhite
A translation of *A Course in Miracles* into plain, everyday
language for anyone seeking inner peace. The companion
volume, *Practicing A Course In Miracles*, offers practical lessons
and mentoring.
Paperback: 978-1-84694-319-5 ebook: 978-1-84694-642-4

Rising in Love
My Wild and Crazy Ride to Here and Now, with Amma, the
Hugging Saint
Ram Das Batchelder
Rising in Love conveys an author's extraordinary journey of
spiritual awakening with the Guru, Amma.
Paperback: 978-1-78279-687-9 ebook: 978-1-78279-686-2

Thinker's Guide to God
Peter Vardy
An introduction to key issues in the philosophy of religion.
Paperback: 978-1-90381-622-6

Your Simple Path
Find happiness in every step
Ian Tucker
A guide to helping us reconnect with what is really important
in our lives.
Paperback: 978-1-78279-349-6 ebook: 978-1-78279-348-9

365 Days of Wisdom
Daily Messages To Inspire You Through The Year
Dadi Janki
Daily messages which cool the mind, warm the heart and guide
you along your journey.
Paperback: 978-1-84694-863-3 ebook: 978-1-84694-864-0

Body of Wisdom
Women's Spiritual Power and How it Serves
Hilary Hart
Bringing together the dreams and experiences of women across
the world with today's most visionary spiritual teachers.
Paperback: 978-1-78099-696-7 ebook: 978-1-78099-695-0

Dying to Be Free
From Enforced Secrecy to Near Death to True Transformation
Hannah Robinson
After an unexpected accident and near-death experience,
Hannah Robinson found herself radically transforming her life,
while a remarkable new insight altered her relationship with
her father, a practising Catholic priest.
Paperback: 978-1-78535-254-6 ebook: 978-1-78535-255-3

The Ecology of the Soul
A Manual of Peace, Power and Personal Growth for Real People
in the Real World
Aidan Walker
Balance your own inner Ecology of the Soul to regain your
natural state of peace, power and wellbeing.
Paperback: 978-1-78279-850-7 ebook: 978-1-78279-849-1

Not I, Not other than I
The Life and Teachings of Russel Williams
Steve Taylor, Russel Williams
The miraculous life and inspiring teachings of one of the
World's greatest living Sages.
Paperback: 978-1-78279-729-6 ebook: 978-1-78279-728-9

On the Other Side of Love
A Woman's Unconventional Journey Towards Wisdom
Muriel Maufroy
When life has lost all meaning, what do you do?
Paperback: 978-1-78535-281-2 ebook: 978-1-78535-282-9

Practicing A Course In Miracles
A translation of the Workbook in plain language, with
mentor's notes
Elizabeth A. Cronkhite
The practical second and third volumes of The Plain-Language
A Course In Miracles.
Paperback: 978-1-84694-403-1 ebook: 978-1-78099-072-9

Quantum Bliss
The Quantum Mechanics of Happiness, Abundance, and Health
George S. Mentz
Quantum Bliss is the breakthrough summary of success and spirituality secrets that customers have been waiting for.
Paperback: 978-1-78535-203-4 ebook: 978-1-78535-204-1

The Upside Down Mountain
Mags MacKean
A must-read for anyone weary of chasing success and happiness – one woman's inspirational journey swapping the uphill slog for the downhill slope.
Paperback: 978-1-78535-171-6 ebook: 978-1-78535-172-3

Your Personal Tuning Fork
The Endocrine System
Deborah Bates
Discover your body's health secret, the endocrine system, and 'twang' your way to sustainable health!
Paperback: 978-1-84694-503-8 ebook: 978-1-78099-697-4

Readers of ebooks can buy or view any of these bestsellers by clicking on the live link in the title. Most titles are published in paperback and as an ebook. Paperbacks are available in traditional bookshops. Both print and ebook formats are available online.

Find more titles and sign up to our readers' newsletter at http://www.johnhuntpublishing.com/mind-body-spirit

Follow us on Facebook at https://www.facebook.com/OBooks/ and Twitter at https://twitter.com/obooks